Social Work and Global Mental Health

This book presents respected experts, researchers, and clinicians providing the latest developments in social work knowledge and research. It discusses the latest in mental health research, information on violence, trauma and resilience, and social policies. Different mental health and social work approaches from around the world are examined in detail, including holistic, ethnopsychiatric, and interventions that place emphasis on recovery, empowerment, and social inclusion. This superb selection of presentations—taken from the 4th International Conference on Social Work in Health and Mental Health held in Quebec, Canada in 2004—comprehensively examines the theme of how social work can contribute to the development of a world that values compassion and solidarity.

The volume offers a unique opportunity for practitioners, researchers, and others in the field to explore respected experts' experiences and research which can spark further development of knowledge that can ultimately enrich humanity as a whole. This timely resource springs from the emerging tradition of the sharing of knowledge, an idea now deeply rooted in the international community of social workers in the areas of health and mental health. This volume is extensively referenced and includes figures and tables to clearly detail information.

This book is enlightening reading for practitioners, administrators, educators, researchers, and students of social work.

This book was published as a special issue of *Social Work in Mental Health*.

Myreille St-Onge and **Serge Dumont** are affiliated with the School of Social Work, Laval University, Quebec, Canada.

Social Work and Global Mental Health

Research and Practice Perspectives

Edited by Myreille St-Onge and Serge Dumont

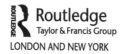
Routledge
Taylor & Francis Group

LONDON AND NEW YORK

First published 2009 by Routledge
2 Park Square, Milton Park, Abingdon, Oxon, OX14 4RN

Simultaneously published in the USA and Canada
by Routledge
270 Madison Avenue, New York, NY 10016

Routledge is an imprint of the Taylor & Francis Group, an informa business

© 2009 Edited by Myreille St-Onge and Serge Dumont

Typeset in Times by Value Chain, India
Printed and bound by CPI Antony Rowe, Chippenham, Wiltshire

British Library Cataloguing in Publication Data
A catalogue record for this book is available from the British Library

ISBN10: 0-7890-3709-2 (hbk)
ISBN10: 0-7890-3710-6 (pbk)
ISBN13: 978-0-7890-3709-1 (hbk)
ISBN13: 978-0-7890-3710-7 (pbk)

CONTENTS

Notes on Contributors

Sandra Blayone is affiliated with Lakeridge Health Corporation, Ontario, Canada.

Jeff Capobianco and Kathy Reynolds are affiliated with the Washtenaw Community Health Organization, Ypsilanti, Michigan, USA.

Normand Carpentier is a Researcher, Institut universitaire de gériatrie de Montréal, and Adjunct researcher, Department of Sociology, University of Montreal, Quebec, Canada.

Cecilia L. W. Chan, PhD, is a Professor at the Department of Social Work and Social Administration of the University of Hong Kong. She is a pioneer in applying Chinese medicine principles and traditional holistic health practices in psychosocial intervention, and, for that, developed the Eastern body-mind-spirit approach. Her current research areas are psychosocial oncology and behavioral health.

Debbie Chan is affiliated with Lakeridge Health Corporation, Ontario, Canada.

Celia H. Y. Chan, MSW, RSW, is a Teaching Consultant at the Centre on Behavioral Health of the University of Hong Kong. Her clinical and research interest is in the application of the Eastern body-mind-spirit approach in infertility counseling.

Neena Chappell is Canada Research Chair in Social Gerontology and Professor, Centre on Aging and Department of Sociology, University of Victoria, Victoria, British Columbia, Canada.

Michèle Clément is a Researcher, GRIOSE-SM, and Adjunct Professor, Department of Anthropology, Laval University, Quebec, Canada.

David Cohen is a Professor at the School of Social Work, Robert Stempel College of Public Health, Florida International University, Miami, Florida, USA.

Lee Crothers is affiliated with ORYGEN Youth Health, Parkville, Victoria, Australia.

Bernadette Dallaire is Associate Professor, School of Social Work, Laval University, and Researcher, Mental Health Research Group on Social Integration and Service Organization and Evaluation (GRIOSE-SM), Quebec Health and Social Services Centre, Quebec, Canada.

Marty Dewees and Lisa K. Lax are affiliated with the Department of Social Work, University of Vermont, Burlington, Vermont, USA.

Kathy Fitzsimmons is affiliated with Lakeridge Health Corporation, Ontario, Canada.

Karen Fletcher is affiliated with ORYGEN Youth Health, Parkville, Victoria, Australia.

Sheila Gallagher is affiliated with Lakeridge Health Corporation, Ontario, Canada.

Baruch Greenwald and Oshrit Ben-Ari are affiliated with Holocaust Survivor Home, Beer Yaakov Mental Health Center, Beer Yaakov, Israel.

Cate Groufsky is affiliated with ORYGEN Youth Health, Parkville, Victoria, Australia.

Catherine Humphreys is a senior lecturer in the School of Health and Social Studies, University of Warwick, UK.

Batya Hyman is an Associate Professor in the Department of Social Work, Salisbury University, Salisbury, Maryland.

Carol Irizarry is affiliated with the School of Social Administration and Social Work, Flinders University, Adelaide, Australia.

Dori Laub is affiliated with the Department of Psychiatry, Yale University, New Haven, Connecticut, USA.

Wendy Leaitch is affiliated with Lakeridge Health Corporation, Ontario, Canada.

Pamela P. Y. Leung, PhD, is a Teaching Consultant of the Centre on Behavioral Health at the University of Hong Kong. She pioneered the integrated body-mind-spirit group intervention for cancer patients in Hong Kong with Professor Cecilia Chan. Her clinical and research interest is in the integration of Eastern philosophy and the body-mind-spirit integrative approach.

Michael McCubbin is a Researcher, GRIOSE-SM, and Adjunct Professor, Faculty of Nursing Sciences, Laval University, Quebec, Canada.

Edward J. Mullen is Willma and Albert Musher Chair Professor, Columbia University School of Social Work, New York, USA.

David Neal is affiliated with the University of Michigan Health System, Ann Arbor, Michigan, USA.

S. M. Ng, BHSc (Chinese Medicine), MSc (Psychiatric Social Work), PhD, is Assistant Professor and Clinical Coordinator at the Centre on Behavioral Health of the University of Hong Kong. His research area is the application of Chinese medicine and traditional Chinese philosophies in mental health practice.

Simon Nudds is affiliated with ORYGEN Youth Health, Parkville, Victoria, Australia.

Sandra Radovini is affiliated with ORYGEN Youth Health, Parkville, Victoria, Australia.

Victoria Ryall is affiliated with ORYGEN Youth Health, Parkville, Victoria, Australia.

Mary C. Ruffolo and Sue Ann Savas are affiliated with the University of Michigan, School of Social Work, Ann Arbor, Michigan, USA.

Carsten Schley is affiliated with ORYGEN Youth Health, Parkville, Victoria, Australia.

Janki Shankar is affiliated with the School of Humanities and Social Sciences, Charles Stuart University, Wagga Wagga, New South Wales, Australia.

Phyllis Solomon is Professor of Social Work, School of Social Policy and Practice and Department of Psychiatry, School of Medicine, University of Pennsylvania, Philadelphia, USA.

Myreille St-Onge and Serge Dumont are affiliated with the School of Social Work, Laval University, Quebec, Canada.

Rael D. Strous is affiliated with Beer Yaakov Mental Health Center, Beer Yaakov, Israel.

Marie-Rosaire Kalanga Wa Tshisekedi is a social worker affiliated with the Outpatient Psychiatry Unit at Hôpital Jean-Talon, Montreal, Canada.

Nancy Veals is affiliated with Lakeridge Health Corporation, Ontario, Canada.

Nancy Wilkinson is affiliated with Lakeridge Health Corporation, Ontario, Canada.

Josephine K. Y. Yau, M.Phil. (I/O Psychology), M.S.Sc. (Psychology), is a Research Coordinator at the Centre on Behavioral Health of the University of Hong Kong. Her research areas are psychosocial intervention evaluation and health scale development and validation.

INTRODUCTION

Social Work and the Development of a More Compassionate World: Experiences and Knowledge to Share

Myreille St-Onge, PhD
Serge Dumont, PhD

In May 2004, the city of Quebec welcomed nearly 800 delegates from 40 countries and five continents within the scope of the 4th International Conference on Social Work in Health and Mental Health. Hosted by the Laval University School of Social Work and the Social Work Department of the Hôtel-Dieu-de-Lévis Hospital, this event took place under the umbrella theme: *Social work and the development of a more compassionate world; experiences and knowledge to share.*

This fourth major gathering has confirmed the emergence of a tradition that is deeply rooted in the international community of social workers working in the areas of health and mental health. Although they are all extremely committed to the various highly specialized fields in which they work, they are bound by a real need to meet with their counterparts to share experiences and further the development of knowledge. They are especially aware that illnesses and mental disorders currently afflicting individuals, their families, and their communities are signs of social inequalities and the current imbalance between human beings and their environment. The fight to alleviate human suffering and the causes and consequences of illnesses and mental disorders thus enriches humanity as a whole. The Fourth International Conference on Social Work in Health and Mental Health provided them with the precious opportunity to reflect together on how social work can contribute to the development of a world that values compassion and solidarity.

The scientific program was structured so as to maximize the sharing of knowledge and views within each area of interest, with the hope of stimulating the emergence of new partnerships. Conference objectives were to:

- Offer a unique occasion to promote the development of knowledge and practices in health and mental health care.
- Foster convergence among creative, leading-edge actors in research and development related to the social aspects of health and mental health.
- Encourage the formation of international partnerships to promote the development of research and training in health care and mental health care.
- Offer graduate students in social work an opportunity to expand their professional network by establishing valuable contacts with colleagues, researchers and clinicians from many regions around the world.

Holding this event made it possible to bring together, under the same theme, internationally renowned speakers and experienced experts, as well as researchers, clinicians, and graduate students from different countries of the world, thus contributing to the reinforcement of collaborative links and dissemination of new knowledge, as well as increasing research capacity within the field of health and mental health.

The quality of the communications was ensured through the presence of internationally renowned speakers providing feature addresses, plenary speeches and satellite symposiums. A scientific committee comprised of 93 members assessed nearly 800 abstracts regarding their innovation and their contribution to the development of knowledge. Five hundred participants were invited to speak or to present poster communications. The Conference themes were addressed by 21 keynote speakers (5 feature addresses and 16 plenary speeches). Moreover, within the scope of the conference's main theme, seven subthemes were addressed through satellite symposiums: social policies, mental health, violence, aging, HIV-AIDS, cancer, and mobility of populations and mobility of health related knowledge.

Of these feature addresses, plenary speeches, and communications, 69 were submitted to be considered for publication. Over the following year, these manuscripts were reviewed by external reviewers. As the guest editors we are proud to offer two special issues, one in *Social Work in Health Care* as well as another in *Social Work in Mental Health*. This current special issue of *Social Work in Mental Health* includes a keynote address, one grand plenary speech, five plenary speeches from the satellite symposia and nine original articles. The issue is comprised of three sections: 1) mental health research, 2) violence, trauma, and resilience; and 3) social policies.

MENTAL HEALTH RESEARCH IN SOCIAL WORK

Mental Health Services Research

The current special issue of *Social Work in Mental Health* opens with an article by Phyllis Solomon which discusses mental health services research for psychiatrically disabled adults from a historical perspective. As she points out, "the relevance of mental health services research is central to social workers in the U.S., as they are the most prevalent providers of mental health care." This situation also holds for Canada and is likely true of other western countries as well. Phyllis Solomon's studies have followed the psychiatric deinstitutionalization movement as well as the development of Community Support Programs in the U.S. that have enabled the elaboration of interventions focusing on psychiatric rehabilitation whose strategies are oriented toward the double objective of client skill development and environmental resources development. Among her research orientations, she has conducted studies on the intersection of mental health and criminal justice systems within the scope of the assessment of the PACT (Program for Assertive Community Treatment) model. The results of her works have shed light on an increased risk of re-incarceration among clients whose follow-up focused quasi-exclusively on monitoring, without offering intensive rehabilitation interventions. Phyllis Solomon has also oriented her studies toward the field of emerging practices in mental health, particularly consumer-operated services, including the provision of mental health services by consumers. The results of this original research—including one of the few randomized studies on this topic—has demonstrated that consumers are as effective as nonconsumers for offering intensive case management services. Finally, another theme of Phyllis Solomon's work relates to support needs for families of psychiatrically disabled people. Among the studies she has conducted in this area, she compared two educational approaches for families: a group family education intervention and an individual family consultation intervention. In her conclusion, the author encourages us, as well as the President of the New Freedom Commission on Mental Health, to transform "the [mental] health system to one that is consumer and family centered and recovery-oriented."

Mary C. Ruffolo and her colleagues Savas, Neal, Capobianco, and Reynolds base their works on those of this same commission recommending the adoption of interventions in respect to best practices for improving the quality of life of consumers and their families living with a serious mental disorder. Within this optic, this article describes a case study implementing multiple family psychoeducation groups (MFG) in the community that are supported by consensus building and decision-making processes. In this study, they formed three community planning groups, two of which included both consumer and family group representatives. The works of these committees led to the development of a MGF logic model to provide support for their implementation and to favor necessary organizational changes. Three MGF pilot projects were thus conducted, to which they added an assessment process. They conclude by highlighting important challenges that need to be addressed and make recommendations for the implementation of evidence-based practice.

Critical Thinking About Psychotropic Medication

In his plenary speech, reported in the current special issue, David Cohen raises fundamental questions regarding the development of knowledge related to psychotropic medication. Cohen presents evidence of the very modest effects of these medications in relation to their generalized use and the trust that several actors within the mental health field have in them. In fact, the World Health Organization (WHO) reports an increase in distress around the world and predicts that by 2020, depression will be the second leading cause of morbidity after cardiovascular diseases. Cohen makes troubling observations regarding studies conducted on psychotropic medication, such as conflicts of interest with pharmaceutical companies and systematic manipulation of results. Cohen raises the central issue as to whether social workers are adequately trained to critically reflect on the use and misuse of medication. A review of 58 Masters in Social Work (MSW) programs in the U.S. revealed students' lack of exposure to critical views with respect to medication treatment and other key topics such as the reliability and validity of psychiatric diagnoses. One should not lose sight of the fact that "knowledge about medications is socially constructed and extremely receptive to the influence of money and power." Within this optic, encouraging consumers to generate formal first-person accounts of their experiences with medication, as David Cohen suggests, may help to re-establish a certain balance between the professionals who suggest compliance with medication treatment and the people directly concerned with their effects.

Holistic Model in Health and Mental Health Social Work

As mentioned by Cecilia Chan and her colleagues in their report, social work in health and mental health "is heavily influenced by Western medicine that focused on [illnesses and disabilities]." It is known that strict recourse to the biomedical model is not sufficient to favor the recovery of people with either mental or physical health problems. In this sense, Chinese medicine, which is based on a holistic perspective and on syndromatic diagnosis as the basis of intervention formulation, places emphasis on ways to favor self-healing among individuals using a multi-model intervention approach. One of the holistic model postulates presented by Chan and her colleagues is that all spheres of human life are interconnected and form a whole. The goal of psychosocial intervention based on this model is to induce changes in all of these systems for a new balance within the person. Chan and her colleagues present examples of their multi-model intervention approach in support of their standpoint.

Critical Approach to Pedagogy in Mental Health

The fact that social workers represent the largest group of professionals in the field of mental health "should render social work's voice in mental health as unique, with a clear sense of identity and an abiding commitment to its legacy of social justice, human rights, and advocacy." However, Marty Dewees and Lisa Lax raise our awareness, in their article, of the risk that many social workers take in adopting a biomedical position by forming their psychosocial diagnoses using the DSM-IV-TR. Within this context, how can one intervene among marginalized populations while not losing sight of social work values, as well as those of justice and the defense of rights? How can one avoid medicalizing social problems such as oppression and racism? Within a critical pedagogy perspective, Dewees and Lax place emphasis on the importance of integrating several discourses into social work teaching that social workers encounter in their professional lives. As such, they propose the teaching of three contents representative of discourse in mental health: the DSM, the theory behind its application from both individual conceptualizations and contextual perspectives, and the importance of understanding his or her epistemological standpoint as a social worker acting within a given society and culture. They conclude by offering pedagogical examples addressing the dimensions of multilingual content and the processes of dialogic critique they considered.

Services for Immigrants

In her paper, Marie-Rosaire Kalanga Wa Thsisekedi describes an ethnopsychiatric approach for immigrants and their families. This approach is used in the psychiatry department of the Jean-Talon hospital in Montreal in the province of Quebec. The intervention program they have developed is inspired by the model developed by French psychoanalyst Tobie Nathan. This program takes into account the cultural diversity of communities with their own knowledge of health and disease. Within this intervention model, inspired by traditional societies, a circular group format is used as a means to solve problems. The author concludes by presenting essential principles on which this approach for immigrants, caregivers, and institutions is based.

Services for Elderly People

In her article, Neena Chappell addresses the issue that while many health problems increase with age, perception of well-being and mental health tends, on the contrary, to improve with age, regardless of socioeconomic status and gender. Within this perspective, Chappell calls upon social workers to take this phenomenon into account by focusing their interventions on a holistic care and health promotion model for elderly people. She cites some models that have recently been elaborated, including the Expanded Chronic Care Model, which combines population health promotion interventions with proven chronic health problem treatments. The author concludes by describing the key role that social workers can play in promoting health among elderly people.

Bernadette Dallaire and her colleagues McCubbin, Carpentier, and Clément address, more particularly, social representations shared by social practitioners about elderly people with severe mental disorders. They point out the sometimes pessimistic attitude that practitioners have regarding the prognosis of these problems among elderly people. They address the importance of interventions using a psychosocial approach that places emphasis on recovery, empowerment, and social inclusion of elderly people with severe mental disorders, while mentioning obstacles to the implementation of such an approach within mental health systems.

Intensive Outreach Services for Young People

Victoria Ryall and her colleagues from ORYGEN Youth Health in Victoria, Australia describe in their article five theories on which they based the development of their intervention model, the Intensive Mobile Youth Outreach Service (IMYOS). This program targets youth aged 12 to 25 years who have complex needs and mental health problems. This population also has difficulty adhering to a traditional treatment model. Their program targets the integration of services for youths and their families, as well as within the system. The majority of the young IMYOS clients have a history of trauma and abuse within their family; within this perspective, the application of attachment theory, trauma theory, and family systems theory is appropriate in order to optimize the assistance offered to these youths. The authors illustrate their intervention with a case history in which the integration of these different theories is demonstrated.

Hospital-Based Group Psychotherapy

Kathy Fitzsimmons and her colleagues from Lakeridge Health Corporation in Ontario, Canada present the results of a study examining a group therapy among 92 adults who completed a mental health day center program in a general hospital. Based on the Young Schema Questionnaire created by Jeffrey Young's team, from the Cognitive Therapy Center in New York, this 6-week group therapy aims to assist clients in making changes in their life patterns in order to decrease depression and anxiety symptoms. The study had a double objective: (1) identify the frequency with which the participants adopted each of the 15 schemas and (2) measure changes in these schemas throughout therapy. Results show that the therapy, which uses a cognitive-behavioral framework including interventions involving communication skills and self-expression, as well as skill and self-esteem development, is effective. Participants had significantly improved in 8 of the 15 schemas at the end of treatment. The authors conclude by pointing out the importance of assessing whether these post-treatment changes are long-term.

VIOLENCE, TRAUMA, AND RESILIENCE

As stated by Cathy Humphrey, there is a strong link between domestic violence and mental health problems among women. In her article, she describes the experiences of women who are victims of spousal violence within the mental health system, where it seems as though the focal point is placed on mental health problems rather than on the violence to which they are victims. This lack of recognition of the violence these women experience unfortunately leads to a form of collusion with the abuser, who often accuses their partners of being "crazy." Accordingly, "contact with the mental health system has the potential to be either inadequate or damaging [from the women's perspective] when the effects of violence and abuse are minimised or rendered invisible." Cathy Humphrey raises new issues that emerge from studies she has conducted with her colleagues regarding the fact that violence is now recognized within the mainstream of statutory services. For example, in the UK, "there are now a raft of new domestic violence policies covering every government department." It is also recognized that spousal violence represents a serious threat to the mental health of the women and children who are victims of this violence. While this tendency to formally recognize violence is accompanied by a greater professionalization of services, she sheds light on how the services offered by women from the voluntary sector have contributed and continue to contribute to the emotional recovery of women experiencing violence. Women working within this sector have always placed an emphasis on essential notions: mutual assistance and recognition of the fact that the violence against women is, above all, a social and political problem. Commitment to this wider agenda to support women is a significant challenge that health professionals must undertake.

In her article, Batya Hyman explores more specifically the link between the violence experience by lesbian women and their mental health. For Hyman, "the mental health of lesbian women is shaped with the unique intersection of violence across the lifespan with the trauma of living in a heterosexist society." The results of studies she has reviewed regarding nonsexual physical violence agree that the incidence of this type of violence is similar for both lesbian and heterosexual women. However, the results diverge regarding sexual violence, with certain studies reporting a greater incidence among lesbian women, while others obtaining similar rates. Furthermore, she reveals a greater incidence of victimization among young lesbian women from their parents and at school. In regards to the link between the violence suffered and mental health problems, studies indicate a much greater proportion of suicide attempts among young lesbian women than among young heterosexuals. The author concludes by pointing out the importance of conducting more studies among young lesbians, as she believes that in the future, young women will reveal their homosexual orientation at a younger age and thus expose themselves to a greater vulnerability in heterosexist school environments.

In her article, Carol Irizarry describes the creation of the group process developed by Flinders University of South Australia School of Social Work, the *Loss and Grief Centre*, to assist women who were placed in the Goodwood Orphanage in Adelaide, Australia between the ages of 5 and 15 following agreements between Australian and British governments to make young British orphans immigrate to Australia following the Second World War. She describes the progress of these women across the activities that they participated through the *Loss and Grief Centre* that led to public recognition of the trauma and grief they experienced as children. These activities, accomplished within a context of mutual assistance, favored the development of resilience in these women.

In Israel, a significant number of hospitalized patients in long-stay psychiatric hospitals are Holocaust survivors. Although these patients do not respond to neuroleptic treatment, most have received a diagnosis of schizophrenia without recognition of the possibility that they are in a state of posttraumatic stress. The goal of the study reported by Baruch Greenwald and his colleagues Ben-Ari, Strous, and Laub was to assess the effect of the use of content analysis of testimonies on video tape as a therapeutic tool among these people. Baruch and his colleagues present three of the testimonies they gathered among 26 people, while placing an emphasis on the reconstruction of their experience. This therapeutic tool not only led to new avenues of expression among people who had become almost mute, but also enabled personnel to better understand their history and develop relationships with them.

SOCIAL POLICIES

Within the context of challenges that public health problems and demographic changes pose for social work, Edward Mullen addresses new developments in evidence-based social policies as a promising strategy of knowledge use aiming to improve the population's physical and mental health state. For Edward Mullen, recourse to this type of rigorous policy elaboration strategies is not at all incompatible with the construction of a more compassionate and just world. Knowledge is a powerful vector for change. Its absence, on the contrary, "can undercut human development and cripple the formulation of intelligent social policies." The field of mental health seems particularly vulnerable to the formulation of social policies that are not based on an in-depth knowledge of the variables at stake. Mullen addresses a series of obstacles that must be overcome to ensure that research is effectively used to guide stakeholders and practitioners in order to establish an informed evidence-based practice. Although this approach is promising, Mullen points out the danger of recourse to this type of research for partisan policy purposes and warns us that "the betterment of social policies has not yet been realized. So we need to be critical about how this innovation will be used and what its outcomes for human development will be in the long run."

Janki Shankar addresses social reforms, particularly with regard to income and employment for people with disabilities, which took place in Australia following the election of a Liberal Coalition Government in 1996. He reviews three recent social policy reforms that, according to him, had a negative impact on the employment of people with psychiatric disabilities. For Shankar "current policies will not only diminish their chances of employment, but will also reduce their chances of recovery." He places emphasis on the policy of mutual obligation, whose objective goes against recovery principles and does not take into consideration research results that demonstrate the number of environmental obstacles that people with psychiatric disabilities must face. Shankar concludes by pointing out that success in seeking employment does not uniquely depend upon the person, but rather on a common effort between individuals and organizations. However, the Australian liberal government reforms are based on competition, economic efficacy, and financial incentives, which leaves little room for people suffering from several mental health problems.

The 4th International Conference in Social Work in Health and Mental Health held in Quebec in May 2004 aimed to significantly contribute to the development of knowledge and practices in social work in health and mental health care within a solidarity enhancement perspective. During the conference, new partnerships emerged between representatives from northern and southern countries. A critical review of the North-South relationships allowed us to recognize the limits of the approaches traditionally adopted in the field of humanitarian aid and developmental assistance. Indeed, politically targeted assistance of some donor countries and paternalist attitude, which unfortunately characterize North-South relations, should make room for cooperation-based initiatives and real partnerships that favor local community participation that respects cultural differences Our initiatives will be successful if we respect human rights and dignity, the underlying values of social work.

The series of articles presented in this issue of *Social Work in Mental Health* offer readers an overview of the wealth of the scientific content of the 4th International Conference and the challenges these issues pose for social work. As guest editors for this special issue, it is with pleasure and pride that we invite you to read on.

SECTION I: MENTAL HEALTH RESEARCH IN SOCIAL WORK

Mental Health Services Research and Its Impact on Social Work Practice with Adults Who Have Severe Mental Illness

Phyllis Solomon, PhD

Mental health services research formally was established in 1956 with amendments to the U.S. National Mental Health Act (NIMH, 1991). The roots of the research domain are in investigations that examined the public psychiatric hospitalization, from admission to care within the facility, and finally, to discharge (Hohmann, 1999; Mechanic, 1989). As the nature of care for adults with severe mental illness (SMI) has grown more complex, so too has the research. But the purpose of this research has remained steadfastly focused on ensuring the most effective care for those suffering from severe psychiatric disorders, with the ultimate goal of improving the quality of life of those affected by these disorders as well as their family caregivers (Hohmann, 1999). Consistent with this purpose the U.S. Department of Health and Human Services issued a plan in 1991 titled *Caring for People with Severe Mental Disorders: A National Plan of Research to Improve Services.* Two more recent reports assessing the status of care for persons with mental illness also issued by the U.S. federal government have called for research in this domain in order to transform the mental health system of care nationally, *The President's New Freedom Commission on Mental Health (2003) and Mental Health: A Report of the Surgeon General (1999).* The Surgeon General's Report noted the "importance of a solid research base for every mental health and mental illness intervention," for "establishing mental health policy on the basis of good intentions alone can make bad situations worse" (p. viii). In this presentation we will examine what some of the accomplishments of this research domain have been and where it needs to go in the future.

The relevance of mental health services research is central to social workers in the U.S., because they are the most prevalent professional providers of mental health care, even more so than psychiatrists and psychologists. Although these mental health service positions may be case managers, family educators, or other service providers, these positions are often held by social workers, but may be filled by individuals trained in other professions as well. The significance of this research to social work will be demonstrated as this report: first, defines and delineates this research domain; second, discusses services and services research for adults with SMI from an historical perspective; and finally, suggests future research directions to ensure the most effective service provision for this very vulnerable population. I will use some of my own research to illustrate particular points.

DEFINING AND DELINEATING SERVICES RESEARCH

Services research investigations examine "a continuum of complexity" from service programs to organizations to mental health service delivery systems to the intersection of various systems with mental health such as social welfare and criminal justice (Hargreaves & Shumway, 1989). As in social work, services research deals with all levels of service intervention strategies, from macro, mezzo, and micro levels. The importance of this area of research was recognized by The U.S. Federal government in 1992 legislation that required the National Institutes of Mental Health, Drug Abuse, and Alcohol Abuse & Alcoholism to expend 15% of their budgets on health services research. This legislation included the following definition for health services research, "endeavors that study the impact of the organization, financing and management of health services on the quality, cost, access to and outcomes of care" (Federal Register, section 409, 1992).

The U.S. National Plan of 1991 previously referred to, further delineated mental health services research into two categories of research, Service Systems and Clinical Services Research. Service systems investigations focus on the macro and mezzo levels by examining organization, financing, administration, and integration of mental health services. This research focuses on service delivery systems and the organizations that comprise these systems. Clinical services research deals with the micro level by researching the process, quality of care, and effectiveness of services and programs (Attkisson et al., 1992; Steinwachs et al., 1992).

HISTORICAL CONTEXT OF SERVICES RESEARCH

With the process of deinstitutionalization, care was no longer confined to psychiatric institutions. Consequently, there was a growing recognition of the need for a diversity of supports and services for persons who were affected by this policy. By the late 1970s the U.S. National Institute of Mental Health had established the Community Support Program (CSP), which developed the Community Support System model of care that recognized that treatment in and of itself was insufficient and that an array of life supports and rehabilitation services was needed (Stroul, 1993).

Psychiatric rehabilitation—a central orientation of this model of care—refers to a diversity of psychosocial service interventions that are directed at changing the skills and/or environmental supports of adults

with SMI (Flexer & Solomon, 1993). The practice of psychiatric rehabilitation is extremely consistent with social work practice in that the
two intervention strategies employed are client skill development and
environmental resource development (Anthony & Liberman, 1986).
Like social work, psychiatric rehabilitation is very value-based in
believing in client self-determination and empowerment and building on
a client's personal strengths by assisting the client in learning coping
strategies to manage the symptoms of the illness and the deficits that
result and in developing a supportive environment in which the client
can function at his/her optimal level (Hughes, 1994; Sands & Solomon,
2001). Psychiatric rehabilitative service interventions include vocational, residential, social/recreational, educational, and case management (Rutman, 1994). Much of psychiatric rehabilitation was initially
provided (from the late 40s to the late 70s) by psychosocial rehabilitation centers that were very much influenced by group work practitioners. Psychiatric rehabilitation evolved from the clubhouse programs
(Mueser et al., 1997). Therefore, psychiatric rehabilitation has been
closely aligned with the consumer self-help movement, as the first
clubhouse program, Fountain House in New York City, was established
by consumers (Mueser et al., 1997).

JUSTIFYING THE NEED FOR PSYCHIATRIC
REHABILITATION FOR DISCHARGED
PSYCHIATRIC PATIENTS

Psychiatric rehabilitation for persons with SMI has been central to
much of my research. When I was deinstitutionalized along with the
patients in 1974, this experience directed my research interest into the
service system arena to determine the access and community service utilization of patients leaving the state psychiatric hospitals. The study that
I designed based on the conceptualization of the Community Support
System model tracked 600 patients for a period of one year, from their
discharge from two psychiatric receiving hospitals through their experiences with the diversity of agencies that comprised the service delivery
system. These service agencies included county welfare department, local
bureau of vocational rehabilitation, social security office, community
mental health centers, specialized community psychiatric programs (e.g., a
psychosocial agency), a residential work program, and group residential
facilities.

The study participants were patients who had numerous and lengthy hospitalizations, yet they received very little in terms of mental health services in the community. Almost three quarters made contact with agencies within the year or prior to readmission, but many received only about two hours of services a month. Further, most did not receive rehabilitative services, but rather medication management, some broker case management, and public financial assistance. Thus, we noted that the system was not geared to improving the level of social functioning of this client population. We recommended the need for a more creative and aggressive approach to vocational rehabilitation, increased use of psychosocial rehabilitation services, the need to address substance abuse problems, and to collaborate with families and consumers in responding to the needs of the population (Solomon, Gordon, & Davis, 1984a&b; 1983). The study findings foreshadowed much of what have been and continue to be the issues for the past two decades in serving this population. Interviewing in depth 60 randomly selected clients from the 600, we found that these clients had the same desires as the rest of us: they wanted a job, a home, and significant others in their lives.

In the closing paragraph of the book published on the study findings, we reported an incident that occurred at the time we were recruiting the study sample, which is quoted in the following:

> A woman patient stood nearby as one of the research assistants attempted to secure consent from another patient for participation in the study. The bystander apparently did not want to be left out. With the sardonic, yet offbeat touch characteristics of many patients, she called out. "Don't pass me over. If you polish me up, I might just be the Hope Diamond." (Solomon et al., 1984a, p. 185)

The sense of hope for individuals with psychiatric disability and belief in their capabilities to grow and change has been a theme throughout much of my research. The one thing in the patient's quote that today I would take issue with is providers not polishing her up, but working with her to acquire the skills and resources for her to polish herself up. The idea is to do *with* clients, not *for* clients, although it is too frequently easier to do for clients, rather than to teach. These are again seen in another study I undertook to assess the barriers to community placement of patients from an extended psychiatric care facility (Solomon, Beck, & Gordon, 1988a&b; Solomon & Gintoli, 1989). These themes are consistent with social work and psychiatric rehabilitation values and approach to service provision and demonstrate further the need for a rehabilitation orientation to servicing this client population (Solomon, 1986-87; Solomon, & Davis, 1986; Solomon, Davis, & Gordon, 1984a).

DEMONSTRATING FURTHER THE NEED FOR REHABILITATION: THE INTERSECTION OF MENTAL HEALTH AND THE CRIMINAL JUSTICE SYSTEMS

As deinstitutionalization progressed, adults with SMI were observed in other human service delivery systems, the homeless shelter system, the welfare system, and more recently in the child welfare system, and the criminal justice system. In response to this population being homeless and in the criminal justice system, in 1989 I designed a clinical service intervention study to assess the effectiveness of a program, entitled the Program for Assertive Community Treatment (PACT) developed for discharged psychiatric patients in Madison, Wisconsin and found to be an effective alternative to hospitalization (Stein and Test, 1980; 1985).

The study was a randomized trial in which adults with SMI leaving jail who were homeless were randomly assigned to one of three conditions: PACT, individual intensive forensic case managers (an existing service), or the usual community mental health system of care. PACT is a self-contained service program delivered by a team of providers, including a psychiatrist, a nurse, case managers, and other specialized providers contingent on the characteristics of target population. Staff to client ratios is very low, usually 1 to 10. The team provides intensive supports, skill teaching, and assistance with environmental supports. Given the nature of the PACT program, the study hypotheses were that those assigned to PACT team would have improved psychosocial functioning, clinical, and quality of life outcomes, including more stable housing, more support system members, and fewer interactions with the criminal justice system than either of the other two conditions, and further, the forensic individual case managers' clients would have better outcomes than the usual system of care. We found that there were no differences among the three conditions with regard to any of these outcomes. However, although not statistically significant, there was a tendency for those receiving PACT to have a greater chance of being reincarcerated than the other two conditions. Overall 46% were reincarcerated at least once within the year of follow-up, with 60% of the PACT clients being reincarcerated, 40% of the intensive forensic case management, and 36% of those receiving usual care (Solomon & Draine, 1995a).

These findings required an explanation, as they were certainly of clinical significance. In further exploration we found that the PACT case managers were working very closely with the criminal justice system. Prior to the clients being released from jail, case managers would go with clients to court for their hearing and would request the judge to place specific stipulations on the clients remaining in the community, such as taking prescribed medication and keeping appointments with the case manager. If the client did not adhere to these stipulations, the case managers worked with the probation and parole officers to technically violate the client. Consequently, the client would be reincarcerated on a technical violation. We found that the PACT case managers were essentially monitoring the clients, they were an extra pair of eyes for probation and parole officers, and therefore, were more likely to observe any violations made by the clients (Solomon & Draine, 1995a).

Two lessons learned from the results of this study were: a lack of fidelity to an intervention can be detrimental for clients and that monitoring without also providing rehabilitation can produce negative consequences for clients. It also seemed that some clients might be returning to jail for treatment purposes, rather than because of criminal activity. The jail from which study participants were coming had a well-developed mental health program, a 65-bed acute inpatient psychiatric program, and an ambulatory psychiatric program. At same time the involuntary commitment procedure in the community imposed very restrictive criteria for hospital admission. Therefore, if clients were not adherent to their medication regime and as a consequence had an exacerbation of their illness, it was easier for case managers to obtain a technical violation of their stipulations with subsequent incarceration than to obtain admission to a psychiatric hospital.

This phenomenon led me to conduct another study that assessed the use of incarceration as a treatment alternative. This study was designed to assess the criminalization hypothesis, that individuals with mental illness enter the criminal justice system due to a lack of access to mental health treatment (Solomon, Draine, & Marcus, 2002). In order to accomplish this objective adults with SMI who were on probation and parole were followed from the point of intake in the psychiatric probation/parole units for 15 months or to reincarceration, whichever occurred first. The primary study focus was to examine the extent to which mental health treatment and adherence explained technical charges as opposed to new criminal charges. The idea was that mental health treatment would prevent the need for future use of jail for treatment purposes. The major findings were that the receipt of intensive case management was associated with reincarceration for technical violations, and negative orientation toward engagement in mental health services was associated with new criminal charges. With these results we again interpreted that intensive monitoring of client behaviors without the provision of rehabilitation to improve their skills and functioning places these clients at greater risk for incarceration. It did not appear that a lack of treatment alternatives was endangering these clients to return to jail.

Another study that I was involved in compared jail diversion services and an in-jail treatment with follow-up services for persons with SMI and substance abuse to determine if diversion reduced an individual's involvement with the criminal justice system. Again monitoring without rehabilitation resulted in negative consequences for the clients, with contact with probation/parole officers resulting in greater likelihood of rearrest (Blank, Draine, & Solomon, 2003).

RESEARCH ON CLINICAL SERVICE INTERVENTIONS

In response to deinstitutionalization and the need for rehabilitation interventions for adults with SMI, a number of innovative clinical service programs were developed to meet the rehabilitation needs of this population. Much of the impetus for the promotion of clinical service interventions that were rehabilitation oriented came from the federal government's Community Support Program (CSP). In the 80s, CSP promoted and funded innovative rehabilitation service interventions, along with small-scale evaluations, which were considered service demonstration projects. Eventually, by the late 80s and early 90s, CSP moved from funding these service demonstration projects to more rigorous research demonstration projects. For the most part, these were randomized trials to determine the effectiveness of clinical service interventions. These funding and promotion efforts greatly contributed to the development of effective clinical service interventions for adults with SMI. Over time there was increasing recognition of the need to assess the fidelity of these service interventions and not merely examine the effectiveness of the interventions. Clinical service intervention research now employs both quantitative and qualitative methodologies, to assess the process of the implementation of the intervention along with the outcomes. To ensure integrity, clinical service interventions have moved to the development of manuals on the structure, principles and procedures for implementation. For example, PACT now has a manual that was commissioned and is sold by the National Alliance for the Mentally Ill, a family advocacy organization (Allness & Knoedler, 1999).

As a result of these service effectiveness studies, there are now a limited number of rehabilitation interventions that are considered evidence-based practice for adults with SMI, particularly for those with schizophrenia. Evidence-based practice as defined by the Institute of Medicine is "the integration of best-researched evidence and clinical expertise with patient values" (as cited in President's Commission Report, 2003, p. 68). "[R]esearch strongly supports the use of specific medications prescribed in specific ways as well as the use of psychosocial interventions such as supported employment, various approaches to illness self-management, family psychoeducation, case management based on the principles of assertive community treatment, and substance abuse treatment that is integrated with mental health treatment" (Torrey et al., 2001, p. 45). The President's New Freedom Commission reiterated the need to support implementation of these same evidence-based practices and also included cognitive and interpersonal therapies for depression. In addition, the Commission Report noted that the mental health field has also documented emerging best practices, "treatments and services that are promising but less thoroughly documented than evidence-based practices" (p. 45). These emerging practices include consumer operated services, jail diversion and community re-entry programs, and trauma-specific interventions. However, one of the major problems is that these evidence-based practices as well as emerging best practices are not widely offered in routine mental health practice settings, and as result few individuals with SMI actually benefit from them. To assist in wider use of these effective interventions, researchers are in the process of developing toolkits to promote the consistent delivery of these intervention practices (Torrey et al, 2001).

My own research has contributed more in the area of these emerging practices, as another major theme of my research has been the capability of consumers to engage in a fulfilling and productive life, including providing mental health services for other consumers. In 1989 in collaboration with consumers of the local mental health association and governmental officials in the Pennsylvania state Office of Mental Health, we designed a randomized trial of consumer-delivered intensive case management service as compared to nonconsumer-delivered intensive case management service funded by CSP. Case managers provided assertive outreach to clients where they lived, worked, and recreated, offering supports and assistance in obtaining services and teaching clients how to manage and adapt to their illness. We hypothesized that clients receiving services delivered by consumer providers would have clinical, psychosocial, and quality of life outcomes as positive as those receiving services from nonconsumer providers.

The idea of consumers having the capability of delivering mental health services to others with similar illnesses was not very widely accepted at the time. We feared that the review committee that assessed the merit of grant applications would not score the application high enough for the proposed study to be funded because of the investigation's lack of feasibility. We therefore designed the consumer intervention to have one member of the team be a nonconsumer provider. Over the course of the implementation of the research, the consumer team became all consumers. The proposed hypothesis was supported by the research, i.e., there were no differences in clinical, psychosocial, or quality of life outcomes for clients served by the consumer and nonconsumer team. Thus, consumer case managers were as effective in delivering case management services as nonconsumers (Solomon & Draine, 1995b&c). This study remains as one of a very few randomized studies on the topic of consumer-provided services (Solomon, 2004; Solomon & Draine, 2001). Consumer-provided services remain an emerging best practice because only a limited number of studies testing the effectiveness of consumer-provided services have employed the scientific gold standard of experimental design.

Another theme of my work is the need to provide supports to family caregivers of adults with SMI. In the early 90s in collaboration with a family member and a recovering family therapist (as she calls herself because she found that she had to unlearn much of what she was taught in her graduate program in family therapy in order to work with families of adults with SMI), a clinical service effectiveness study of a family education program was designed and funded by CSP. This was a randomized investigation of two family educational interventions developed by these two collaborators, a group family education intervention and an individual family consultation intervention. The group educational workshop consisted of 10 weekly two-hour sessions that provided information and methods for developing coping skills. Each session was facilitated by a family member and a professional provider. The family consultation, an individualized educational approach, was provided for a minimum of

6 hours and maximum of 15 hours over the course of three months. The consultant functioned as an educator and advisor, and assisted the family in setting their goals around issues and concerns regarding their ill family member and then helping to achieve these goals. The service was delivered in person or by phone, with the initial session being in person. These two educational approaches were compared with each other and with a waitlist control. The hypothesis for study was that those families receiving the educational interventions would have a decrease in subjective burden, grief, and stress; an improvement in adaptive coping with and self efficacy and mastery in managing their relatives' illness; and increased social support at termination of the intervention. This hypothesis was partially supported — the family interventions were helpful in increasing the self-efficacy of family members, but the group intervention was only effective for those who had not engaged in family advocacy (Solomon, Draine, Mannion, & Meisel, 1996; 1997). Although only partially supported, it needs to be kept in mind that these were relatively limited interventions for families who had been living with their relatives' illness on average for 17 years. The positive finding demonstrates the strength of the intervention: it is amazing that it had an effect at all under these circumstances. The service providers found being involved in the research to be a humbling experience. They truly believed in the effectiveness of their interventions and very much wanted to demonstrate their efficacy with hard evidence. They approached me as a researcher to work with them. The results did direct them to make modifications in their services, which they feel have improved their service (Mannion et al., 1997).

Another aspect of this study was to assess the secondary benefit that the ill relative of these families might receive as a result of the participation by the families in an education program. We hypothesized that brief family education interventions would have a positive impact on clinical outcomes for the ill relatives whose family members participated in the interventions. The study found that ill relatives whose families participated in the educational interventions did improve their attitudes toward medication compliance (Solomon et al., 1996). This illustrates the potential of family education, as one explanation for the positive outcomes for family educational interventions generally is improved medication compliance (Solomon et al., 1997).

Family education is not considered an evidenced-based practice because of limited research. However, collaboration of providers working with families of adults with SMI has also been promoted by practice guidelines issued by the American Psychiatric Association (1997) and other expert groups (Frances, Docherty, & Kahn, 1996). In collaboration with the recovering family therapist mentioned earlier and other colleagues, a community action grant was obtained from the U.S. Federal agency, Substance Abuse and Mental Health Services Administration, to develop a manual and train providers in the incorporation of family consultation into routine care for adults with SMI. Family education is not the same as family psychoeducation (which is an evidence-based practice), as family education is education with no requirement of treatment for either the family or ill relative, whereas psychoeducation does require the ill relative to be in treatment and taking prescribed medication (Solomon, 1996).

Currently, I'm involved in a HIV prevention intervention for adults with SMI and substance abuse disorders. Although this is a population at greater risk for this illness than the general population, there has been little done in terms of routinely educating this population about risks and prevention of HIV/AIDS and other sexually transmitted diseases. This intervention is delivered by case managers.

I am also currently the Co-Principal Investigator for a National Disability Rehabilitation Research grant for a research and training center on community integration for adults with SMI. Specifically, I'm involved in research on conceptualization and measurement of the community integration construct and in the development of an intervention to be delivered by case managers to enhance the social networks of adults with SMI. I am also evaluating a mental health workforce training program in cultural competency. This evaluation has demonstrated the need for more conceptual and measurement work for the construct of cultural competency.

FUTURE DIRECTIONS OF SERVICES RESEARCH FOR ADULTS WITH SEVERE MENTAL ILLNESS

Despite the growing evidence in the arena of service interventions for adults with SMI, there is limited use of these interventions in routine care. There is a need to increase our knowledge with regard to transmission and receptivity of new clinical service interventions by providers. The lack of knowledge in this domain has been recognized by the U.S. National Institute of Mental Health, resulting in the issuance of a specific program announcement to encourage research on this topic. Further, research on service interventions needs to continue to be vigorously pursued, as we have not been successful in achieving the important outcomes for many in this population, including stable and decent housing, higher functioning, and employment. Also, those service interventions that are emerging best practices are areas of considerable importance and therefore require additional research. However, much of mental health service research on the implementation of evidence based practice has focused on program structure, such as caseload size, staffing, frequency of team meetings, but it is also essential for research investigations to delve into micro areas of service interventions.

Anthony (2003a & b) has well articulated this point by noting that "evidence based practice initiative has overlooked in these program descriptions the ingredients of the helping process that occur within each practice" (p. 2). Increasing our understanding of these "human interactive processes" are essential to improving client outcomes in conjunction with the implementation of evidence based practices. For example, it has been suggested that a lack of positive outcomes for social functioning with Assertive Community Treatment (ACT) programs may be the result of an inattention to social skill training (Mueser et al., 1998). Increased understanding of these processes may offer direction for how we train providers in these evidence practices such that they will be receptive to implementing them. As a social worker and current president of the International Association of Psychiatric Rehabilitation Services, Anita Pernell-Arnold, noted in response to the findings of the tracking study regarding the need for psychiatric rehabilitation for patients discharged from the psychiatric hospitals reported on earlier, "just as the clients do not like to fail, neither do the providers." Providers do what they feel most comfortable and successful doing. Even if they do implement an innovative service after training, over time they slip back into their old ways of functioning.

The President's New Freedom Commission recommended transforming the nation's mental health system to one that is consumer and family centered and recovery-oriented. In this report, recovery was defined as "the process in which people are able to live, work, learn, and participate fully in their communities. For some individuals, recovery is the ability to live a fulfilling and productive life despite a disability. For others, recovery implies the reduction or complete remission of symptoms." (p. 5) A recovery orientation is a significant shift away from the medical model that focuses on symptom reduction toward one that is far more encompassing of the individuals client's goals, which may not be concerned with symptoms. Consequently, a recovery orientation recognizes that a client's goals may differ from those of the clinician. A recovery process is a very personal one, and one that respects the wishes of the client and offers hope to the client (Solomon & Stanhope, 2004). To implement this recovery orientation, examining these human interactive processes is essential. For example, there is a need to determine the strategies, such as coercion or limit setting, that providers employ in their interactions with particular types of clients under specific circumstances. Similarly, alliances between providers and clients is another area in need of further research. There has been limited research in this domain with clients with SMI, because for too long many providers believed that this population was incapable of forming relationships with others. I and a few other investigators have conducted research on the alliances between providers and clients with SMI on clinical and psychosocial outcomes and found that positive alliances do result in improved outcomes (Draine & Solomon, 1996; Solomon, Draine, & Delaney, 1995).

In a recent article entitled "Recovery: The Heart and Soul of Treatment" by Townsend, a social worker, and Glasser (2003), they reported on a client who dreamed of becoming an astronaut, but his case manager wouldn't take it seriously. Further, when the client refused to indicate another goal, the case manager reported in the progress notes that the client was "uncooperative and delusional." The client went on to work with another case manager who also perceived this interest as nothing but a pipe dream. Finally, another case manager respected the client's dreams and asked the client to investigate what it would take to become an astronaut. The client found that becoming an astronaut was far more work than he wanted. However, "his interest in space was real and important to him" (p. 84). The case manager worked with him to obtain employment with a company that worked in the space industry. This story very much represents a recovery orientation for working with clients and how respecting a client's wishes and interests and believing in the client's capabilities can produce successful outcomes for both the client and the provider. A recovery orientation is a human interactive process that requires research that can provide direction for training and intervention development.

Another goal of the New Freedom Commission was to ensure that culturally competent mental health services are delivered. Cultural competent services were defined as "the delivery of services that are responsive to the cultural concerns of racial and ethnic minority groups, including their language, histories, traditions, beliefs, and values" (p. 52). This is an essential area of research, because it is not clear to what extent evidence-based practices are effective with cultural diverse groups. Again, culturally competent providers incorporate a cultural orientation into their service provision as with the recovery orientation.

Both recovery and cultural competency requires work on conceptualizing and operationalizing these constructs. The methodological approaches to examining these interactive processes require some creative thinking with regard to how we go about researching these concepts and processes. Just as time and resources were put into conducting randomized studies of service intervention and developing fidelity assessments of implementation, we now need to proceed to the next step of researching inside the black box of service interventions.

Research into these human interactive processes needs to extend beyond providers collaborating with their clients, to collaboration with family members. Mental health service researchers who investigate services for adults with SMI also need to examine the impact of the environmental context on these processes. Environmental context includes micro, mezzo, and macro environments, such as the organization and its culture, the inter-relationship between organizations, as well as the community in which the service is delivered. There has been limited research in the human services on these variables and their impact on services. The one exemplar of the impact of these variables on human service delivery has been the work of Charles Glisson, a social worker, who has found that organizational climate impacts the quality of services in the child welfare system (Glisson & Hemmelgarn, 1998).

SUMMARY AND CONCLUSIONS

In the last two decades, mental health services research has come a long way in helping to improve services for adults with SMI. But we must continue to keep up the momentum that has been started. As is evident by the future research directions that are sketched out above, there is much work to be done. Without a concerted effort to broaden the array of interventions, to further refine these evidence-based practice interventions to ensure that they are responsive to a recovery orientation and to a diversity of cultural groups, and to increase our understanding of how providers can be assisted and supported in working with clients and families, we can't expect our clients to shine like the hope diamond or we as providers to feel successful.

REFERENCES

Allness, D., & Knoedler, W. (1999). *The PACT Model of Community-Based Treatment for Persons with Severe and Persistent Mental Illness: A Manual for PACT Start-Up.* Arlington, VA: National Alliance for Mental Illness.

American Psychiatric Association (1997). American Psychiatric Association Practice Guidelines for the Treatment of Patients with Schizophrenia. *American Journal of Psychiatry, 154* (Apr. suppl.), 1–63.

Anthony, W. (2003a). Editorial. *Psychiatric Rehabilitation Journal, 27,* 1–2.

Anthony, W. (2003b). Studying evidence-based process, not practices. *Psychiatric Services, 54,* 7.

Anthony, W., Liberman, R. (1986). The practice of psychiatric rehabilitation: Historical, conceptual, and research base. *Schizophrenia Bulletin, 12,* 542–559.

Attkisson, C., Cook, J., Karno, M., Lehman, M., McGlashan, T., Meltzer, H., O'Cconnor, M., Richardson, D., Rosenblatt, A., Wells, K., Williams, J., & Hohmann, A. (1992). Clinical services research. *Schizophrenia Bulletin, 18,* 561–626.

Blank, A., Draine, J., & Solomon, P. (Nov. 2003). Diversion vs. Jail Services: Enhancing Surveillance? American Society of Criminology Annual Conference, Denver, CO.

Department of Health and Human Services. (1999). *Mental Health: A Report of the Surgeon General.* Rockville, MD: DHHS.

Department of Health and Human Services. (2003). *New Freedom Commission on Mental Health: Achieving the Promise: Transforming Mental Health Care in America. Final Report* (No. DHHS pub. No. SMA-03-3832). Rockville, MD: DHHS.

Draine, J., & Solomon, P. (1996). Case management alliance with clients in an older cohort. *Community Mental Health Journal, 32,* 125–134.

Flexer, R., & Solomon, P. (1993). Introduction. In Flexer, R., Solomon, P. (eds.) *Psychiatric Rehabilitation in Practice.* Boston: Andover Medical Publishers.

Frances, A., Docherty, J., & Kahn, D. (1996). Expert consensus guideline series: Treatment of Schizophrenia. *Journal of Clinical Psychiatry, 57:* 1–58.

Glisson, C., & Hemmelgarn, A. (1998). The effects of organizational climate and interorganizational coordination on the quality and outcomes of children's service system. *Child Abuse and Neglect, 22,* 401–421.

Hargreaves, W., & Shumway, M. (1989). Effectiveness of services for the severely mentally ill. In Taub, C., Mechanic, D., & Hohmann, A. (eds.): *The Future of Mental Health Services Research.* Rockville, MD: U.S. Dept. of Health and Human Services.

Hohmann, A. (1999). A contextual model for clinical mental health effectiveness research. *Mental Health Services Research, 2,* 83–91.

Hughes, R. (1994). Psychiatric rehabilitation: An essential health service for people with serious and persistent mental illness. In IAPSRS Publication Committteee (ed.): *An Introduction to Psychiatric Rehabilitation.* Columbia, MD: International Association of Psychosocial Rehabilitation Services.

Mannion, E., Draine, J., Solomon, P., & Meisel, M. (1997). Applying research on family education about mental illness to development of a relatives' group consultation model. *Community Mental health Journal, 33,* 555–569.

Mechanic, D. (1989). The evolution of mental health services and mental health services research. In Taub, C., Mechanic, D., Hohmann, A. (eds.): *The Future of Mental Health Services Research*. Rockville, MD: U.S. Dept. of Health and Human Services.

Mueser, K. T., Bond, G., Drake, R., & Resnick, S. (1998). Models of community care for severe mental illness: A review of research on case management. *Schizophrenia Bulletin, 24*, 37–74.

National Institute of Mental Health (NIMH). (1991) *Caring for People with Severe Mental Disorders: A National Plan of Research to Improve Services*. DHHS Pub. No. (ADM) 91–1762. Washington, D.C.:DHHS.

Rutman, I. (1994). What is psychiatric rehabilitation? In IAPSRS Publication Committeee (eds.): *Introduction to Psychiatric Rehabilitation*. Columbia, MD: IAPSRS.

Sands, R., Solomon, P. (2001). Social work curriculum and psychiatric rehabilitation. *Psychiatric Rehabilitation Skills, 5*, 405–413.

Solomon, P. (2004). Peer support/peer provider services: Underlying processes, benefits, and critical ingredients. *Psychiatric Rehabilitation Journal, 27*, 392–401.

Solomon, P. (1996). Moving from psychoeducation to family education for families of adults with serious mental illness. *Psychiatric Services, 47*, 1364–1370.

Solomon, P. (1986–87). Receipt of aftercare services by problem types: psychiatric, psychiatric/substance abuse, and substance abuse. *Psychiatric Quarterly, 58*, 180–188.

Solomon, P., Beck, S., & Gordon, B. (1988a). Family members' perspective on psychiatric hospitalization and discharge. *Community Mental Health Journal, 24*, 121–130.

Solomon, P., Beck, S., & Gordon, B. (1988b). A comparison of perspectives on discharge of extended-care facility clients: Views of families, hospital staff, community mental health workers and clients. *Administration in Mental Health, 15*, 166–174.

Solomon, P., & Davis, J. (1985). Meeting community service needs of discharged psychiatric patients. *Psychiatric Quarterly, 57*, 11–17.

Solomon, P., & Davis, J. (1986). The effects of alcohol abuse among the new chronically mentally ill. *Social Work in Health Care, 11*, 65–74.

Solomon, P., Davis, J., & Gordon, B. (1984). Discharged state hospital patients' characteristics and use of aftercare: Effect on community tenure. *American Journal of Psychiatry, 141*, 1566–1570.

Solomon, P., & Draine, J. (2001). The state of knowledge of the effectiveness of consumer provided services. *Psychiatric Rehabilitation Journal, 25*, 20–27.

Solomon, P., & Draine, J. (1995b). One year outcomes of a randomized trial of case management with seriously mentally ill clients leaving jail. *Evaluation Review, 19*, 256–273.

Solomon, P., & Draine, J. (1995c). The efficacy of a consumer case management team: Two year outcomes of a randomized trial. *Journal of Mental Health Administration. 22*, 135–146.

Solomon, P., & Draine, J. (1995a). One year outcomes of a randomized trial of consumer case management. *Evaluation and Program Planning. 18*, 117–127.

Solomon, P., Draine, J., & Delaney, M.A. (1995). The working alliance and consumer case management. *Journal of Mental Health Administration, 22*, 126–134.

Solomon, P., Draine, J., Mannion, E., & Meisel, M. (1997). Effectiveness of two models of brief family education: Retaining gains of family members of adults with serious mental illness. *American Journal of Orthopsychiatry, 67*, 177–186.

Solomon, P., Draine, J., Mannion, E., & Meisel, M. (1996). The impact of individualized consultation and group workshop family education interventions on ill relative outcomes. *Journal of Nervous and Mental Disease, 184*, 252–254.

Solomon, P., Draine, J., Mannion, E., & Meisel, M. (1996). Impact of brief family psychoeducation on self efficacy. *Schizophrenia Bulletin, 22*, 41–50.

Solomon, P., Draine, J., & Marcus, S. (2002). Predicting incarceration of clients of a psychiatric probation and parole service. *Psychiatric Services. 53*, 50–56.

Solomon, P., & Gintoli, G. (1989). Research as an impetus for change in a state psychiatric hospital. *Journal of Mental Health Administration, 16*, 247–251.

Solomon, P., Gordon, B., & Davis, J. (1984a). *Community Services to Discharges Psychiatric Patients*. Springfield, IL: Charles C. Thomas.

Solomon, P., Gordon, B., & Davis, J. (1984b). Discharged state hospital patients' characteristics and use of aftercare: Effect on community tenure. *American Journal of Psychiatry, 141*, 1566–1570.

Solomon, P., Gordon, B., & Davis, J. (1983). An assessment of aftercare services within a community mental health system. *Psychosocial Rehabilitation Journal, VII*, 33–39.

Solomon, P., & Stanhope, V. (2004). Recovery: Expanding the vision of evidence-based practice. *Brief Treatment and Crisis Intervention, 4*, 311–321.

Stein, L., & Test, M.A. (1980). Alternative to mental hospital treatment: I. Conceptual model treatment program and clinical evaluation. *Archives of General Psychiatry. 37*, 392–397.

Stein, L., & Test, M. A. (1985). *The Evolution of the Training in Community Living Model*. San Francisco: Jossey-Bass.

Steinwachs, D., Cullum, H., Dorwart, R., Flynn, L., Frank, R., Friedman, M., Herz, M., Mulvey, E., Snowden, L., Test, M.A., Tremaine, L., & Windle, C. (1992). Service systems research. *Schizophrenia Bulletin, 18*, 627–668.

Stroul, B. (1993). Rehabilitation in Community Support Systems. In Flexer, R., Solomon, P. (eds.): *Psychiatric Rehabilitation in Practice*. Boston: Andover Medical Publishers, pp. 45–62.

Torrey, W., Drake, R., Dixon, L., Burns, B., Flynn, L., Rush, A. J., Clark, R., & Kealzker, D. (2001). Implementing evidence-based practices for persons with severe mental illnesses, *Psychiatric Services, 52*, 45–50.

Townsend, W., & Glasser, N. (2003). Recovery: The heart and soul of treatment. *Psychiatric Rehabilitation Journal, 27*, 83–86.

The Challenges of Implementing an Evidence-Based Practice to Meet Consumer and Family Needs in a Managed Behavioral Health Care Environment

Mary C. Ruffolo, PhD
Sue Ann Savas, MSW
David Neal, MSW
Jeff Capobianco, MS
Kathy Reynolds, MSW

The President's New Freedom Commission on Mental Health (2004) calls for a transformation of the behavioral health care system; interventions are to be guided by best practices, driven by consumers and families, and result in quality of life improvement for consumers and families living with a mental illness. To increase the effectiveness and efficacy of intervention services, models of evidence-based practices

(EBP) have been adopted by many managed behavioral health care organizations. However, efforts to integrate EBP into real world behavioral health care settings often fail to produce the same outcomes that demonstrated positive change for consumers and families in the controlled experimental settings used to establish and test the models (Anthony, Rogers, & Farkas, 2003). Yet, it is no longer acceptable for behavioral health care organizations to plan and develop programs within the mental health service delivery system without being informed by the current research on EBP. Managed behavioral health care organizations are faced with the challenge of adopting, translating and implementing EBP within real world mental health practice environments.

A community-centered model of planning is one approach for introducing, implementing, and adapting the EBP more effectively. This community-centered model is participatory, grounded in best practices, and uses systematic processes for gathering input and conducting evaluations (Wandersman, 2003). Wandersman (2003) identifies three areas that need to be addressed by behavioral health care organizations when considering the adoption of EBP. These areas include: accessibility, credibility, and expectations. In addressing accessibility, Wandersman (2003) suggests that behavioral health care organizations examine if they have the same resources available as the researchers who developed the EBP. When addressing credibility of the EBP, it is important for the behavioral health care organization to determine how different their practice environment is from the research settings where the EBP was developed and tested. Finally, Wandersman (2003) recommends that behavioral health care organizations define their expectations for practice improvements prior to the implementation of EBP.

Similarly, Green (2001) advocates for using a planning process to examine the appropriateness of EBP for the setting and the population. Green (2001) recommends that behavioral health care organizations include systematic input by administrators, practitioners, consumers, and families. Through planning, implementation of EBP, and on-going evaluation of the practice, outcomes are expected to improve for consumers and families. When planning for service system improvements, it is important for behavioral health care organizations to understand that there is no one path to mental health recovery and the processes for one person may be different than for another person (Anthony et al., 2003).

According to Wandersman, Imm, Chinman, and Kaftarian (2000), behavioral health care organizations can increase the probability of achieving positive outcomes by addressing the following: current organizational needs and resources, goals for the target population, how the EBP fits with other programs already being offered, capacity of practitioners to deliver the EBP, integration of measures to ensure fidelity, strategies for evaluating whether the change is working that include consumer and family input, and how the EBP will be sustained over time.

This report will describe how a managed behavioral health care organization used a community-centered model of planning to adopt and implement an evidence-based practice, multiple family psychoeducation groups (MFG) for adults living with schizophrenia and their families. The paper will review a consensus building and decision-making processes used to: (1) develop an implementation plan for adapting the model, including a feasibility assessment to identify existing and needed organizational resources; (2) orient and train clinicians and key community stakeholders; (3) pilot test the EBP; (4) establish an ongoing evaluation plan to monitor fidelity to the model and track outcomes; and (5) develop a plan to sustain the practice. The processes used to engage practitioners, consumers, and families in the development and implementation of the EBP for this community will also be presented. For other communities committed to integrating EBP, the challenges and recommendations for bridging the EBP with a real world practice setting will be outlined.

SETTING AND EVIDENCE-BASED PRACTICE

The managed behavioral health care organization (MBHC) in this study operates as an integrated mental health, substance abuse and physical health care delivery system for Medicaid and indigent consumers in one mid-western county. The MBHC contracts with the county mental health community support and treatment services organization to provide mental health services for persons with serious mental illness. As an organization, the MBHC adopted six core principles to guide their community-centered planning work: consumer and family involvement, comprehensive quality services, community based services, public accountability, integrated care, and involvement of research and medical education. The community-centered planning process described in this paper was facilitated by university-based evaluators.

Built upon the MBHC's commitment to consumer and family involvement, the organization reviewed several EBP models for best fit with their current practice. Based on the results from this review of the research and with input from the local Nation's Voice on Mental Illness (NAMI) chapter, the MBHC organization selected multiple family group psychoeducation (MFG) as the EBP for this community-centered planning process. Current research established family interventions, psychoeducation approaches and specifically MFG as an EBP ready for adoption. Randomized clinical trials have repeatedly demonstrated that family interventions that educate families about mental illness, provide support, and offer training in effective problem-solving and communication, in combination with appropriate pharmacotherapy, reduce one year relapse rates from 40% to a 53% range and improve consumer and family functioning from 2% to a 23% range (Dixon, Adams, & Lucksted, 2000; Lehman, 1999; Dixon & Lehman, 1995, McFarlane et al., 1996, McFarlane et al., 1995). Key elements for successful psychoeducation programs include: being professionally led, being offered as part of the overall treatment package that includes medication, enlisting consumers and families as partners in treatment, and focusing on outcomes (Dixon et al., 2000; McFarlane et al., 2000) In addition, multiple family psychoeducation group outcome studies on clinical and theoretical implications demonstrate that:

- Family intervention is more effective than individual treatment and/ or medication alone.
- Multiple family group approaches are specifically more effective than single family approaches for first-episode and high-risk patients, poor responders to medication, or patients in highly stressed families.
- Multiple family psychoeducation groups result in higher rates of employment and lower morbidity than single family support.
- The benefits of multiple family group increase with time (more than 4 years) (McFarlane, 2002).

Consistent with the core values of the MBHC, this community mental health intervention moves away from a traditional individualized approach to a consumer and family-centered practice approach. The population and the setting used to develop and test the MFG model closely matched the community's target population and service environment. After a preliminary review, administrators reported that organizational resources and the capacity of practitioners to deliver the EBP seemed promising. The community made the commitment to implement multiple family psychoeducation groups. As the lead organization, the MBHC sought and was awarded a SAMHSA funded community action planning grant to further the adoption and implementation of multiple family psychoeducation groups. Consumer, family and provider stakeholders were brought together for dialogue and consensus building sessions to improve services and outcomes for adults with severe mental disorders.

COMMUNITY-CENTERED PLANNING PROCESS

The community-centered planning process was designed to focus on three primary goals: (1) to use community consensus building activities to explore implementation of the Multiple Family Psychoeducation Group (MFG) intervention; (2) to examine organizational resources for Multiple Family Psychoeducation Group (MFG) implementation; and (3) to provide initial training in the MFG model. Regular meetings of two primary community planning groups and one financial/administrative planning group were convened. The MFG Collaborative Planning Group members

(25) represented different consumer groups, family groups, and key clinical and administrative staff from the major organizations that would implement the MFG model within the MBHC network. The focus of the MFG Collaborative Planning Group was to build consensus and develop a logic model and a set of practice principles for the MFG implementation. In addition to examining and articulating the MFG model for the community, the MFG Collaborative Planning Group addressed "readiness for change," organizational and clinical capacity building issues to integrate MFG into the service delivery system. This group met monthly to address their tasks. The second group, Community Cross-system Advisory Group (40 members) consisted of key stakeholders from mental health and physical health organizations, housing, clubhouses, substance abuse programs, and consumer/family groups. The group met every other month and reviewed the consensus building work of the MFG Collaborative Planning Group, addressed system barriers, and identified cross system service changes needed for successfully implementation of the MFG. The financial/administrative group (8 members) included top administrators from MBHC and the primary organizations that serve MBHC consumers. Under a capitated model, MFG is seen an intervention that promotes recovery and is cost effective. Organizational resources needed to support MFG implementation were reviewed, including training needs of staff, supervision issues, role of the psychiatrist, access and funding. The financial/administrative group met periodically at key decision-making points. Members of the evaluation team participated in and observed all of the group decision-making processes.

RESULTS

These three community planning groups examined the multiple needs of adults with severe mental disorders and their families with a special focus on the needs of young adult consumers, African American consumers, women and consumers with co-morbid mental health and substance abuse or physical health issues. The dialogue, consensus building and planning process resulted in the adoption of a community relevant MFG logic model (See Figure 1), a set of common principles of practice to support the implementation effort, and an implementation plan outlining the organizational changes and resources needed to facilitate the implementation of MFG. The process and the documents were evidence of the community's shift to a more culturally sensitive, consumer and family based approach.

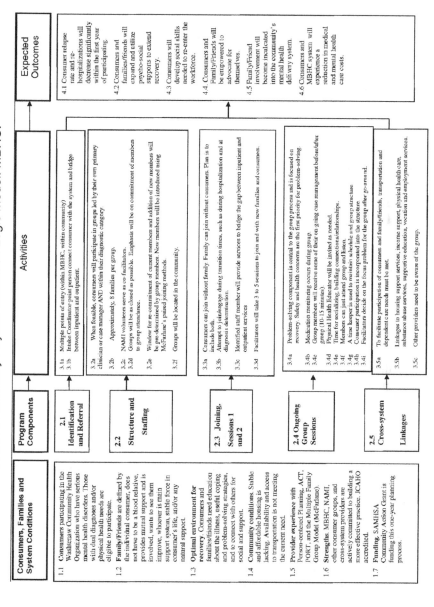

FIGURE 1. Family Psycho-education Logic Model: MBHC.

Early in the community-centered planning process, to facilitate under-standing of the EBP, a 2-day MFG orientation training by the lead researcher and practitioner in this approach was provided to clinicians, consumers/family members, supervisors and managers. A booster session with clinicians and consumers/family MFG co-facilitators was convened six months later to respond to implementation and integration issues, including ongoing supervision needs. Two primary methods were selected to maximize fidelity to the adapted MFG model. These methods included use of the MFG fidelity scales developed by the original researchers of the EBP and on-going supervision/consultation from the developers of MFG for the first year of implementation.

In addition to the community-centered planning activities and training, three MFG pilot groups were implemented to assess the relevance of the model for the community: two of the groups focused on young adult con-sumers and one group included Assertive Community Treatment consum-ers. The pilot groups operated with the tri-leadership model of group facilitation. This model includes one mental health professional, one case manager and one NAMI consumer/family member as MFG group facili-tators. The tri-leadership model is an adaptation of the EBP that reflects the realities of the implementing service organization and the value orien-tation of the MBHC, as well as, the strong advocacy voice of the local NAMI chapter. Process evaluation findings from the pilot groups, indi-cate that consumers and family members found the MFG intervention very helpful, attendance was regular and the problem solving themes were consistent with addressing the challenges of living with a severe mental disorder (See Table 1). In addition, the pilot study findings indi-cated a change in the way consumers and families relate to the mental health service system: most of the intervention work is occurring within the group setting, crisis responses have decreased, medication adherence is strong and hospitalizations/psychiatric emergency service use has decreased.

The evaluation of the community-centered planning process was designed to be transparent, objective, and valued as an integral part of the planning and development process. This evaluation approach was used to facilitate ownership of the process and model problem-solving processes rather than as an externally imposed burden. The evaluation process included conducting pre and post stakeholder interviews (N = 37), summarizing the data from the stakeholder interviews, track-ing attendance at meetings, maintaining meeting notes, administering brief post-session meeting feedback forms to assess the successes and

TABLE 1. Consumer and family/friend feedback (N = 50) from MFG pilot groups

Survey Item	Satisfaction of Respondents
Today I found the group to be helpful to me	82% agree
The group leaders and I agree about the things I will need to do in group to help improve my situation	80% agree
What I am doing in group gives me new ways of looking at my situation	78% agree
I feel the group appreciates me	77% agree
I believe that the group members like me	72% agree
I am confident of the group's ability to help me	72% agree
The group members do not understand what I am trying to accomplish in group	71% do not agree
Members of the group and I are working towards mutually agreed upon goals	70% agree

challenges of the consensus building process, graphic mapping of decision making process prepared after each meeting for use at the next group meeting, and evaluation of the training orientation, the pilot groups, booster sessions and monitoring adherence. All the evaluation results were routinely shared with the planning groups for reflection and refinement of the process.

In order to sustain the EBP, the MBHC made a financial commitment to consumers and families, as well as their provider organizations to continue to support efforts to implement MFG throughout the system. In one concrete way that the MBHC is supporting the sustainability of the EBP is to purchase on-going supervision and consultation from the lead research group for the MFG intervention. The staff and consumers, family members who receive the ongoing supervision after one year will be able to train future community-based group leaders in the MFG model. In addition, a Community Cross-system Advisory Group was established to serve as an ongoing resource and consultation unit to provide oversight of needed services (i.e., physical health care, housing, transportation, vocational/employment) for adults with severe mental disorders and their families using the MFG framework. The MFG intervention is being implemented throughout the organization and new groups are starting monthly.

One of the greatest barriers to implementation of the EBP was addressing the billing services codes at the state level for this practice since the focus was on family and not just the consumer. It is important to address the financial mechanisms early in the process of implementing an EBP.

SUMMARY AND RECOMMENDATIONS

Using a community-centered planning process to bring evidence based interventions into an integrated health care environment is time intensive but it promotes the critical steps necessary for sustainability of the EBP. The community-centered planning process allowed for systematic input from a wide range of stakeholders, addressed the potential barriers to implementation and allowed for the adaptation of the model within the realities of the current system. This approach to organizational change decreased resistance from staff and increased services to families in the organization. Consumers and families were actively involved in all stages from selection of the EBP to the implementation/evaluation of the EBP. The consumers and families had a "decision-making voice" throughout the entire process. In order to maximize consumer and family input in the community-centered planning efforts, it is important to address potential barriers to meeting attendance, such as transportation issues. Regular de-briefing sessions with the consumers and families were also central to the success of this process. Operationalizing the practice guidelines, articulating expectations of the EBP, adapting the EBP to the realities of the community practice and pilot testing the MFG intervention were essential steps. Using on-going supervision with clear practice guidelines, clinicians and consumer/family member co-facilitators were able advocate for needed changes to maintain intervention fidelity. It is critical to not underestimate the importance of addressing work place culture issues in the process of transitioning from one form of clinical practice to a different form of clinical practice that requires maintaining fidelity to EBP guidelines.

Some of the key challenges in using a community-centered planning process is keeping all stakeholders involved in the process, making sure that stakeholders are informed and ready to make decisions at meetings and addressing conflicts that may surface among stakeholders during this process. To address these challenges, it is important to establish rules about how decisions will be made early in the process to minimize stakeholder drop-out and conflict. Communicating with stakeholders through regular newsletters that focus on the community-centered planning progress is another way that stakeholders can stay informed and involved in the process.

The recommendations for adopting of EBP in a managed, behavioral health care environment, includes:

- Using a community-centered planning process that is grounded in consensus building activities will maximizes stakeholder input for decision-making
- Using tools, such as, logic models and practice principles, will facilitate understanding of the EBP and establishes a common theory of change
- Assessing work place culture issues that might facilitate or impede implementation of an EBP.
- Pilot testing of the EBP will allow an organization to assess the fit of the EBP within a service delivery network
- Ongoing process and outcome evaluation of the community-centered planning process as well as the EBP implementation will provide the key stakeholders with feedback for process improvement.

REFERENCES

Anthony, W., Rogers, E.S., & Farkes, M. (2003). Research on evidence-based practices: future directions in an era of recovery. *Community Mental Health Journal 39/2.* 101–114.

Dixon, L., Adams, C., & Lucksted, A. (2000) Update on family psychoeducation for schizophrenia. *Schizophrenia Bulletin, 26*(1), 5–20.

Dixon, L.B. and Lehman, A.F. (1995) Family interventions for schizophrenia. *Schizophrenia Bulletin, 21*(4):631–43.

Green, L. (2001). From research to "best practices" in other settings and populations. *American Journal of Health Behavior, 23*(3), 165–178.

Lehman, A. (1999). Quality of care in mental health: the case of schizophrenia. *Health Affairs, 18*(5), 52–65.

McFarlane, W.T. (2002). *Multifamily Groups in the Treatment of Severe Psychiatric Disorders.* New York: Guilford Press.

McFarlane, W.R., Dushay, R.A., Stastny, P., Deakins, S., & Link, B. (1996). A comparison of two levels of Family Aided Assertive Community Treatment. *Psychiatric Services, 47*, 744–750.

McFarlane, W.R., Dushay, R., Deakins, S., Stastny, P., Lukens, E., Toran, J., & Link, B. (2000). Employment outcomes in Family-Aided Assertive Community Treatment. *American Journal of Orthopsychiatry, 70*(2), 203–214.

McFarlane, W.R., Lukens, E., Link, B., Dushay, R., Deakins, S.A., Newmark, M., Dunne E.J., Horen, B., & Toran, J. (1995) Multiple-family groups and psychoeducation in the treatment of schizophrenia. *Archives of General Psychiatry, 52*(8): 679–87.

Wandersman, A. (2003). Community Science: bridging the gap between science and practice with community-centered models. *American Journal of Community Psychology, 31/3–4*, 227–242.

Wandersman, A., Imm, P., Chinman, M., & Kaftarian, S. (2000). Getting to outcomes: a results-based approach to accountability. *Evaluation and Program Planning, 23*, 389–395.

Needed: Critical Thinking
About Psychiatric Medications

By the late 1980s, biological psychiatry was finally consecrated as the reigning school of thought in mental health (Healy, 2002). Anyone could now confidently attribute deviance, distress, and dysfunction to neurotransmitter imbalances in individual brains, and the bulk of public and private funding for mental health research shifted to support neurobiology and drug treatments. For any psychological affliction in men and women, taking psychotropic drugs became the treatment of first resort. By 2000, 13% of middle-aged women in America reported taking antidepressants (National Center for Health Statistics, 2004).

Despite 50 years of modern psychopharmacology practiced on a large scale, even modest improvements in outcomes of conditions routinely treated with drugs cannot be discerned (Cohen, 1997a; Healy, 1997; Kessler et al., 2003; Research Triangle Institute, 2002; Whitaker, 2002) and some evidence suggests that drugs are making things worse. In a large population study, depressive episodes occurring in antidepressant users were three times more frequent (11% vs. 3.5% incidence) and lasted nearly twice as long (19 weeks vs. 11 weeks) than episodes among depressed nonusers (Patten, 2004). The rate of attempted suicide, for which depression is believed to be the major precursor, shows no robust or overall decline despite the large increase in antidepressant drug treatments (van Praag, 2002). Schizophrenia, the disorder for which antipsychotic drugs have been most exhaustively prescribed since 1954, seems to fare no better. In a meta-analysis of 368 outcome studies spanning 100 years (Hegarty et al., 1994), rates of remission of schizophrenia reached in 1992 a level statistically indistinguishable from that observed in the 1920s, when hydrotherapy was in vogue. Generally, the increase in the use of psychopharmaceuticals does not correlate with indicators of reduced morbidity. Using 1987 (when Prozac was introduced) as a benchmark, Robert Whitaker (personal communication, 2004) estimated that 3.505 million people in the U.S. received Supplemental Security Income or Social Security Disability Income for mental disorders. By 2002, that number had reached 5.77 million (a 64% increase). These findings do not establish that use of medications is sustaining or exacerbating dysfunction, but they suggest that, at least from a population health perspective, use of medications has not reduced dysfunction.

The pharmaceutical industry, meanwhile, became the planet's most profitable (Fortune, 2000). Psychotropic drugs now rank second or third among most prescribed drugs. In 2003, sales of all central nervous system–acting drugs in the United States exceeded $37 billion. That year, world sales of the eight top-selling antidepressants reached $15.7 billion and three psychotropics were among the world's ten top-grossing pharmaceuticals (IMS Health, 2003). One of them, the antipsychotic Zyprexa (olanzapine), had generated $13.5 billion in sales during a mere 6 years on the market.

These numbers and their magnitude help explain why in 2001 eight of the nine largest drug companies spent more on advertising, promotion, and administration ($19 billion in the U.S.) than on research ("New 2001 data shows," 2002). That last staggering sum itself explains why the pharmaceutical industry is undoubtedly the most influential actor in the health and mental health systems today. Its influences "extend to federal regulatory agencies, professional organizations, medical journals, continuing medical education, scientific researchers, media experts, and consumer advocacy organizations" (Antonuccio, Danton, & McClanahan, 2003, p. 1028). Moreover, considering how much money can be made from selling a well-promoted drug that passed the regulatory hurdles to gain market approval, the incentives for this industry to manipulate scientific activities may be irresistible. Recently, so much evidence of such outright manipulation has come to light that mental health professionals who ignore it do so at their own peril, because this evidence is shaking the few scientific foundations of psychiatric drug treatment.

THE LATEST "CRISIS" IN THE MENTAL HEALTH SYSTEM

From about 2001 onward, media and scientific reports have shed unprecedented light on a grave practice undermining public health: drug companies' concealment of unfavorable findings from their clinical drug trials. With negative data censored by sponsors and those who actively or passively help them, published clinical trial reports are not credible. Concealment is widely agreed to occur because the health and mental system are rife with conflicts of interest (Sharav, 2003, 2004), which have grown along with the growth of the pharmaceutical industry and the commercialization of drug research (Arnold & Relman, 2002).

Conflicts of Interest in Government Agencies

Although U.S. Federal regulations generally prohibit the Food and Drug Administration (FDA) from using experts with financial conflicts of interest, the FDA waived that requirement over 800 times between 1998 and 2000, and over half the experts on FDA Advisory Panels had financial ties with the commercial enterprises most affected by the panels' recommendations (Cauchon, 2000). For their part, the National Institutes of Health in 1995 allowed their "scientists to spend unlimited time consulting for outside employers, with no ceiling on the resulting income," according to the *Los Angeles Times* (Wilman, 2004). This policy was rescinded in 2005.

More indicative of an extraordinary slant toward industry, the FDA intervened with a Federal judge's order in August 2002 requiring Glaxo-SmithKline to stop advertising that its antidepressant "Paxil [paroxetine] is non habit forming." Using easily available evidence, the judge had ruled that the commercials were "misleading and created inaccurate expectations about the ease of withdrawal" ("Judge: Paxil ads," 2002). The FDA's own chief counsel—formerly best known for suing the FDA on behalf of the pharmaceutical industry—argued, however, that only the FDA was authorized to decide what should be disclosed in drug advertisements (Kranish, 2002). In October 2002, the British Broadcasting Corporation (BBC) documentary *Panorama* provided compelling "anecdotal" evidence of patients' extreme difficulty in withdrawing from Paxil. The BBC received 67,000 phone calls and 1,500 emails from viewers providing additional evidence of Paxil-induced severe withdrawal symptoms. Shortly thereafter, GlaxoSmithKline revised upward 500-fold its rate of Paxil-induced withdrawal symptoms, from 0.05% to 25% (Medawar & Hardon, 2004).

Illegal Promotional Efforts by Drug Companies

The deceitful promotion of the newer "atypical" antipsychotic drugs among state governments in the U.S. has also been alleged recently, due to a whistleblower's release of internal documents. According to the *New York Times*:

> Since the mid-1990's, a group of drug companies . . . has campaigned to convince state officials that a new generation of drugs . . . is superior to older and much cheaper antipsychotics . . . The campaign has led a dozen states to adopt guidelines for treating schizophrenia that make it hard for doctors to prescribe anything but the new drugs. . . . Ten drug companies chipped in to underwrite the initial effor by Texas state officials to develop the guidelines. Then,

to spread the word, [these] companies paid for meetings around the country at which officials from various states were urged to follow the lead of Texas . . . Sales of the new antipsychotics totaled $6.5 billion [in 2003] . . . [Costs of state Medicaid programs] have ballooned with the adoption of the new drugs. Texas, for example, says it spends about $3,000 a year, on average, for each patient on the new drugs, versus the $250 it spent on the older medication. (Peterson, 2004)

Following another whistleblower's revelations, Pfizer, the world's largest drug company, agreed in May 2004 to pay a fine of $430 million after pleading guilty to a charge of criminal fraud in the illegal promotion of Neurontin (gabapentin), an adjunct anti-seizure drug. Physicians recruited by Pfizer touted Neurontin's wonders for bipolar disorder, migraine, back pain, ADHD, and depression, indications unstudied and unapproved by the Food and Drug Administration. Ninety percent of Neurontin's sales in 2003 ($2.7 billion) were for these off-label indications (Armstrong & Mathews, 2004).

Crude Suppression of Negative Trial Findings

Without the full picture of a drug's performance in a clinical trial, or with an exaggerated picture of a drug's benefits, recommendations for treatment are likely to be erroneous. "Publication bias" has long been criticized as a form of scientific misconduct (Chalmers, 1990), but when journalists investigated suppression of findings from clinical trials involving children on antidepressants, the Attorney General of the State of New York filed a lawsuit in 2004 against GlaxoSmithKline (formerly SmithKline Beecham) for "repeated and persistent fraud by concealing and failing to disclose" that its drug Paxil/Seroxat (paroxetine) did not demonstrate a benefit for youth in clinical trials (Harris, 2004a; Kondro & Sibbald, 2004). The Attorney General charged that at least five studies testing Paxil in youth were conducted, only one study showing mixed efficacy and safety was published, while the negative findings from the four other studies—showing no efficacy and an increase in suicidal ideation—were suppressed. Nearly 900,000 Paxil prescriptions to youth were written in the U.S. in 2002.

GlaxoSmithKline initially responded in its defense that data were not concealed: they were submitted to the FDA and other nations' agencies charged with ensuring the safety and effectiveness of drugs and approving their marketing. However, in April 2004, members of the U.S. Congress had asked FDA officials to explain not only why they had not acted on data in their possession—linking antidepressants to increased suicidal ideation in depressed children—but why they also had forbid the FDA's own principal reviewer from publishing his analysis confirming these risks (Harris, 2004b; Shogren, 2004; Waters, 2004).

That same month, both the *British Medical Journal* and *The Lancet* published meta-analyses of all pediatric selective serotonin reuptake inhibitor (SSRI) clinical trials, which for the first time included the unpublished data obtained from the U.K.'s drug regulatory agency. In this more complete portrait, and in stark contrast to conclusions found in individual trial reports published in American journals, four of five tested drugs showed no or "doubtful" effectiveness but excess adverse effects, over placebo pills (Jureidini et al., 2004; Whittington et al., 2004). The accompanying *Lancet* editorial stated: "The story of research into selective serotonin reuptake inhibitors (SSRI) use in childhood depression is one of confusion, manipulation, and institutional failure" ("Depressing Research," 2004).

Medical Journals as Advertising Pamphlets

Medical journals have been described, even by their own editors, as "an extension of the marketing arm of the pharmaceutical companies" (Smith, 2005). Journal editors are said to "fake a control over their journals which they no longer have" (Fava, 2004, p. 1). Dependent on drug firms for advertising revenues, journals cannot resist publishing reports of randomized controlled trials (RCTs) with which drug companies flood journals because clinicians believe RCTs constitute superior forms of evidence. Many RCTs are industry-sponsored and most conclude that their sponsor's product is superior or equivalent to alternatives. For example, not one of 124 published clinical trials of three atypical antipsychotics sponsored by their manufacturers reported negative results (Procyshyn et al., 2004). Peer review seems largely ineffective: when the *American Journal of Psychiatry* published "the first" RCT of citalopram for youth depression, reporting positive conclusions (Wagner et al., 2004), neither the authors nor the editors mentioned that a previous RCT by the same sponsor had reached *negative* conclusions, but had not been published (Meier, 2004). Journals' task is made more difficult by individual researchers in academia and government who—as in the pediatric Prozac studies funded jointly by Eli Lilly and Company and the

National Institute of Mental Health—sign "secrecy agreements" that withhold essential information about the drugs' effects (Harris, 2003). Smith, former editor of the *British Medical Journal*, believes that only a radical step could reverse journals' growing irrelevance as vehicles of scientific information: Journals should *stop publishing trials*. Instead, they should concentrate on critically evaluating trials.

Medicines Out of Control?

In a detailed case study of the antidepressant fiasco, Medawar and Hardon (2004) conclude with provocative remarks that apply to all psychopharmaceuticals and perhaps to all medications today:

> Are medicines out of control? The question reflects concerns about endemic and pathogenic institutional secrecy; rampant conflicts of interest; systematic manipulation of "scientific" evidence and perversion of understanding; the marginalization of dissenting, inconvenient and unwanted views; official indifference to essential and valuable evidence from patients; the rising dominance of trade imperatives and the sickening promotion of disease awareness; the emphasis on pharmaceutical innovation as the source of health solutions; the size and cost of the Pharmas in relation to their health value; the inadequacy of self-regulation and the lack of democratic accountability—and the consequences of this for health for one and all. (p. 222)

Medawar and Hardon's remarks describe a mental health system completely at odds with its self-defined mission of providing care to suffering "consumers" and scientific guidance to society. The passage recalls previous indictments of previous crises of the mental health system. For social work scholars and practitioners, this should call into question their role in contributing to the dysfunction.

Social Work and Critical Thinking About Psychiatric Drugs

Today, social workers are ubiquitous in mental health settings and many of their tasks relate to medication management, including cajoling, persuading, or coercing clients to follow prescribed drug regimen, and not without ethical unease (Floersch, 2002; Walsh, Farmer, Taylor, & Bentley, 2003). Activities of social workers enable the taking of medications by clients within a mental health service system that essentially revolves around "medication compliance."

Proposing "best practices" for referring clients for psychiatric medication, Bentley, Walsh, and Farmer (2005) urge their colleagues to "avoid appearing as cheerleaders for the pharmaceutical industry" but also "avoid being pessimistic naysayers who discount all rigorous research as biased" (p. 5). Discounting "rigorous research" appears unscientific indeed, but precisely where are social workers to find such research? Are they exposed to authors who describe the systematic debasement of RCTs over the last two decades (Relman & Angell, 2002)? Only the last (Bentley, 2003) of four social work books on psychopharmacology published since 2000 (Austrian, 2000; Dziegielewski & Leon, 2001; Bentley & Walsh, 2001) contains some critical discussion of the role of the pharmaceutical industry in the mental health system, or of biases in information sources on which social workers rely. Analyzing syllabi of 60 graduate social work courses on psychopathology, Lacasse and Gomory (2003) find a single article on negative effects of medication as a recommended reading, in less than 1% of syllabi. They also find a startling reliance on secondary sources rather than primary empirical reports, as recommended readings generally. Persuing *Social Service Abstracts* with the keywords "pharmaceutical industry," I found a single article in a professional social work journal that seems to discuss the topic critically. This evidence suggests that the social work literature on medications virtually *excludes* serious discussion of key sociopolitical issues that might encourage practitioners and students to think critically about psychotropic medications. Generally, as Lacasse and Gomory observe, "There is little evidence that graduate psychopathology courses cover viewpoints other than the most conventional and institutional—that of biomedical psychiatry" (2003, p. 383).

Over the past century, major schools of thought in mental health have overstated their scientific claims to justify obtaining or maintaining political and cultural influence (Fancher, 1995). Key ideas and interventions touted as reform or progress at one moment were later repudiated as misleading or damaging (e.g., Braslow, 1997; Dolnick, 1998; Johnson, 1990). Arguably, the history of mental health care recounts mistakes about mental health care: physical and mental harm caused to ordinary people seeking help from approved experts, therapies, and schools of thought (Diekelmann & Kavanagh, 2002; Illich, 1976; Morgan, 1983). The history of healing confirms healers' capacity to harm, which is the reason for the helping professions' best-known ethical precept, "First, do no harm."

Professionals who understand this history choose carefully which ideas and practices merit their allegiance. This is "critical thinking"—stepping outside conventional ways of viewing something and submitting it to ethical, logical, and historical scrutiny (Gibbs & Gambrill, 1999). Today's conventional idea in mental health—that people behave in ways unapproved or unacceptable because they have something wrong with their genes or brain, a problem that is best fixed with drugs—is just what needs more scrutiny.

The need for social workers to develop a critical perspective on the use of psychiatric drugs is long past due. Unless social workers cease being users of second-hand, nonrigorous, biased studies funded by the industry that gains most from their dissemination, and begin to generate *their own basic knowledge about drugs*, social work's claim to being a full-fledged mental health profession rings hollow. And social workers' practical support for psychotropic drug treatments may be, simply, unethical. Should social workers not join neuroscientists, physicians, epidemiologists, psychologists, consumers, and advertising companies in producing knowledge about drugs?

Today, mostly because of the advent of the Internet and its capacity to give direct voice to individuals, expert knowledge about drugs has to accommodate the voices of individuals in areas that psychopharmacologists have consistently downplayed or denied, such as withdrawal effects (Breggin & Cohen, 1999). Subjective drug effects, part of people's "lived reality," are an obvious point of entry for basic social work research in psychopharmacology (Farmer & Bentley, 2002). In helping encounters, creating spaces for detached evaluations of psychotropic drugs (Cohen, 2003) takes on added importance because of the return, since the 1920s, of direct-to-consumer advertising of prescription drugs, and their current availability to almost anyone via Internet sites, turning medications into consumer products and admen into key intermediaries between people and their medications. From the critical perspective espoused in this article, social workers in this mutating and complex mental health field could also undertake the pressing intellectual task of asking basic questions about psychopharmacology, biological psychiatry, and psychotropic drugs, and testing and refining answers to these questions that resonate with core values of the healing professions and with the principles of scientific inquiry unsullied by economic or narrow professional interests. In the following sections, I ask some of these questions, about biological psychiatry, psychopharmacology, psychotropic drugs, and placebo effects, hoping to offer heuristic comments with some testable elements. A rather more "social" view of medications emerges from these comments, but one that hopefully does justice to the complexity of the phenomena and that indicates several lines of investigation.

Biological Psychiatry and Psychopharmacology: Progress in Mental Healing?

Does the popularity of biological psychiatry rest on its success in providing validated answers to age-old conundrums about mental suffering and healing? Perhaps its popularity rests on the simple facts that many people like to use drugs for reasons that are important to them, and that psychiatry provides culturally acceptable justifications for this use (Fancher, 1995). Using drugs to alter consciousness, to ease pain, to induce sleep or maintain wakefulness are old and universal practices. Biological psychiatry exploits these ordinary desires with a medical/scientific rhetoric, currently that of the "biochemical imbalance." People hear, read, and are taught that psychotropic drugs are prescribed for them because medical science has discovered that their brain functioning is defective, and that drugs "work" by correcting or compensating for these imbalances.

Moncrieff and Cohen (2005) suggest that this view has important weaknesses: (1) it cannot logically justify the use of drugs since all major pathophysiological hypotheses about mental disorders were derived from observed actions of drugs; (2) comparisons between drugs believed to have specific effects in certain conditions and drugs thought to have non-specific effects fail to support it; (3) in clinical trials, outcome measures (i.e., symptom rating scales) for various disorders include items responsive to nonspecific drug effects; (4) studies with healthy volunteers describe characteristic drug-induced states independently of a psychiatric diagnosis; and (5) animal tests show effects with drugs not usually thought of as specific treatments for the conditions modelled by tests.

Reductionist biological explanations (i.e., that schizophrenia results from dopamine overactivity, or that depression results from serotonin underactivity) are commonly presented as scientific facts although none has been demonstrated (Mental Health, 1999). They situate deficiencies deep within individuals, but outside of their control. In this way, they resemble discarded dogmas that mental health practitioners used to espouse fervently, such as the all-powerful but invisible unconscious. We must ask: to what extent do distressed individuals feel *empowered* by viewing themselves as genetically or neurochemically deficient and by remaining on guard for undetectable biochemical imbalances?

Viewed historically, the idea that giving people psychotropic drugs represents an obvious scientific advance over conversation or guidance seems too uncritically accepted. Giving someone in distress something to swallow is a primal custom that resonates with our earliest experiences as powerless infants, and of course that perpetuates what was arguably a substance-rich evolutionary past for the human species (Sullivan & Hagen, 2002). Substance use and substance seeking are human universals. Licit and illicit healers throughout recorded history have used substances to treat ailments, and sufferers have claimed to benefit from substances whether or not medical science could validate the claims (Szasz, 1974).

What are Psychotropic Drugs?

Psychotropic drugs are material substances that are ingested inside the body and, according to current ideas in neurophysiology, exert effects on the brain to alter feeling, behaving, and thinking. Drugs' material properties are essential for any understanding of their effects. Yet much of the significance of drugs in people's lives comes from drugs' power as *symbols*. From an anthropological perspective, drugs might be seen as "charged objects" (like talismans, amulets, or sacraments) laden by humans with powers, hopes, and fears. Certainly, names ascribed to drugs (and then erroneously reified as drug *properties*) confirm the value of this perspective: "antidepressant," "mood stabilizer," "cognition enhancer," and many more. Medications can become triggers for personal change, leading some users to radically reinterpret their very sense of self. From a more sociological perspective, medications are (1) an interface between patients and physicians; (2) tools of social control; (3) causes and consequences of medicalization; (4) reservoirs of badness ("dangerous drugs") or goodness ("approved medications") for mainstream society; and (5) vectors of globalization, given that a few developed countries sell most medicines to the rest of the world (Cohen, McCubbin, Collin, & Perodeau, 2001). In sum, drugs are powerful material objects that interact with our neurophysiology, but they are also socially grounded phenomena that are highly responsive to culture and history, producing "effects" that reverberate within and outside individuals' bodies to shape social relations in families, in groups, in institutions, and in societies.

Drug Effectiveness or Placebo Effects?

Modern medications appear as the ultimate products of rational and bio-technological design. Yet, to establish a drug's therapeutic efficacy, the world's highest scientific and regulatory standards involve comparing it to a pharmacologically *inert* substance, a "placebo." Undoubtedly, this says as much about the power of placebos than the effectiveness of drugs. In re-analyses of the very best clinical trials of seven modern "antidepressants" (submitted to the FDA by manufacturers to gain the drugs' market approval), Kirsch, Moore, Scoboria, and Nichols (2002) showed that about 85% of the improvement in medicated subjects was matched in placebo-treated subjects. This needs restatement: 85% of positive effects that medication-treated adult depressed subjects in a clinical trial attribute to their medications might be achieved merely by giving them a sugar pill and having them believe it *might* be an antidepressant. Even if defined "simply" as the patient's "expectation of recovery," such an effect looms as *hugely* significant, clinically as well as statistically. However, because the placebo is unpretentious and nameless, placebo benefits can be claimed by its competitors. And, instead of investing the resources needed to investigate the power of this vital human capacity for self-repair and its relationship to individuals' places and roles in social contexts, the placebo is often dismissed as amounting to "no treatment" or "nothing." Here is Medawar and Hardon's more "social" view of the placebo effect:

> All sorts of human beliefs, motivations and styles of organisation make medicines work as they seem to do. These factors are typically invisible, go largely unrecognized and have no other name. They go largely incognito. . . . The fact that they have no collective name underlines that their impact is generally unrecognised and therefore poorly understood. Probably the main reason is that the word placebo has come to stand for *all* the non-drug factors that affect treatment outcomes. It does not seem an appropriate word: it does not take into account of many non-pharmacological factors on treatment outcomes . . . (Medawar & Hardon, 2004, p. 175).

The felt effectiveness of a treatment or a medicine has to do not only with the relationship between user and drug or patient and doctor. Doctors and patients' experiences and history, their norms, statuses, and roles, their faith and hope—not to mention suggestion from their peers and from advertising, drug company sponsorship of clinical events, the names given to drugs—must also count as major factors in drug "effectiveness."

Are "Therapeutic" Effects Socially Constructed?

The perception of a drug effect as *therapeutic* depends on human motives within particular social contexts. For example, neuroleptic drugs produce abnormal movements in humans and animals, but how the abnormal movements of psychiatric patients on neuroleptics were initially labeled (or even noticed) and how they were acted upon depended on expectations of clinicians in mid-20th century mental hospitals (Cohen, 1997b). Whether doctors or patients view sedation from a benzodiazepine as as a "therapeutic effect" or an "adverse effect" has nothing to do with the pharmacology of benzodiazepines and everything to do with what doctors and patients are seeking at different times (Cohen & Karsenty, 1998). Whether indifference and lack of initiative in formerly depressed patients taking Prozac is labeled as "improvement" or "frontal lobe damage" depends on how long and how closely the patients and the clinician have been interacting (Hoehn-Saric, Lipsey, & McLeod, 1990; Jacobs & Cohen, 1998). Whether obedience and cognitive overfocusing in a child taking psychostimulants is seen as "effectiveness in reducing off-task behavior" or "an expression of the continuum of stimulant toxicity" depends largely on teachers' expectations of children in a structured classroom.

In sum, "therapeutic" and "adverse" effects of psychotropic drugs do not spring directly from molecules. They refer to judgments made by various interested parties about the *value* of particular drug effects. If this is the case, why certain of these judgments are accepted as "psychopharmacological facts" may depend more on the parties' relative power in the prescription situation than on the validity of their judgments.

Are Licit Drugs Better than Illicit Drugs?

Virtually all illicit psychotropic drugs today—from heroin to cocaine to amphetamines to LSD—were once promoted or prescribed as useful remedies. From a strictly pharmacological point of view, one cannot explain why drugs are available legally or not, considered beneficial or harmful, dispensed only by prescription or sold freely over the counter. Pharmacologically, one cannot account for the different social fates of two classical stimulants with nearly identical neurochemical effects: methylphenidate (Ritalin) and cocaine (Vastag, 2001). Likewise, amphetamines were formally rejected in 1971 by medical and law enforcement authorities internationally. These drugs were described as trapping users into dependence and triggering violence and psychosis after prolonged high-dose use (Grinspoon & Hedblom, 1975). Yet, in 2003 a mixture of three pure amphetamine salts marketed as Adderall was among the drugs on which spending for children in the U.S. exceeded spending for antibiotics (Johnson, 2004).

Many other examples confirm that the fate of a psychotropic drug in society has little to do with its known and predictable effects and much to do with how legal and medical authorities might be affected by its widespread use. To complicate matters, every 15 to 20 years, authorities change their minds about the benefits or dangers of particular substances. The unsettling truth is that licit status, approval by the FDA, promotion by manufacturers, prescription by doctors, and praise by patients do not necessarily indicate what consumers and prescribers might really wish to know about a drug's "safety" or its "effectiveness." Unarguably, future observers will pay scant attention to a drug's institutional approval when assessing how it *actually* impacted those who took it.

CONCLUSION

From the varied perspectives and interests of different professions and disciplines, there are still countless questions to ask about psychiatric drugs and the clinical and social contexts in which their uses are embedded. No guarantee can be given that useful answers will be found. But if something is to be learned from the crisis in the legitimacy of *prescribing psychotropic drugs as medicines* that I and others claim exists today, it is that "problems arise not because [experts] don't know enough, but when they behave as if they do" (Medawar & Hardon, 2004, p. 182).

Biological psychiatry, in an unholy symbiosis with the pharmaceutical industry, has actively promoted the view that people's emotional problems are symptoms of diseases of the body (brain), usually resulting from genetic abnormalities, and has transformed ritualistic substance use into scientific therapy (Fancher, 1995). Public funds and public employees now privilege the availability of drugs over other forms of help and support. The result is that hundreds of social, economic, spiritual, psychological, and educational problems are now treated as *diseases* located inside individuals' bodies, a trend commonly referred to as medicalization (e.g., Conrad & Schneider, 1992). If previous history and systems thinking serves as a guide, such a paradigm shift, though perhaps inevitable, cannot have only positive implications nor can its most important negative consequences be anticipated. Thus, a moral duty of practitioners who wish to avoid harming clients is to scrutinize the clinical paradigms that legitimize their professional power and behavior.

The age of medicalization, like the centuries-old age of faith that preceded it, also carries its share of intellectual mystification, iatrogenic injury, and sociocultural decline. Fully a quarter of the population is implied to be genetically deficient because affected with "diagnosable" or "treatable disorders" (*Mental Health*, 1999). In one of history's strangest social experiments, up to 15% of children in some North American communities are given stimulants and other drugs to make them conform to their schools' and their families' expectations. Long-term psychotropic drug use can be shown to be detrimental for individual brains. Will it be shown to be detrimental for the species' evolutionary capacity (Fukuyama, 2002; Nesse & Berridge, 1997)? In human bodies, families, and groups, drugs banish neither stress nor the principal *sources* of stress, nor do they enhance people's capacity to *cope* with stress—drugs only seem to blunt people's *responses* to stress (Mirowsky & Ross, 2003).

In a free society, people whose lives have been disrupted and traumatized by the slings and arrows of fate can choose to use psychotropic drugs. Obviously, people can derive self-defined benefits from the psychological and behavioral alterations that psychotropic drugs characteristically produce. Precisely *how many* people derive such benefits remains largely unknown, given the paradigmatic emphasis in mental health on drugs as obvious therapeutic advances. For the same reason, it also remains largely undetermined just how temporary or laden with unpleasant surprises might drug-associated benefits be for ordinary individuals in their ordinary circumstances (Jacobs & Cohen, 1998).

In parallel, and just as obviously, healers can choose to follow the time-honored and lucrative tradition of giving drugs or encouraging the use of drugs. However, we now possess sufficient information, some of which I summarized at the beginning of this article, to ask to what extent this healing stance rests on validated science, critical thinking, and genuine patient preference, and to what extent it rests on social pressure and marketing efforts. We can also ask to what extent this stance actually thwarts clinicians' ability to sustain helping relationships (Smith, 2001). And to answer these questions, we cannot simply turn to authorities and secondary sources, but must engage in critical thinking. Not only "facts" but their "conditions of production" must be included in our efforts to advance knowledge and understanding and improve healing. In particular, it hardly seems possible today to use the findings of countless clinical trials in psychopharmacology to enlighten us about the positive psychological effects of drugs or to inform us accurately about drugs' potential risks. More specifically, this large body of clinical research might be completely useless to suggest ideal conditions for drug use in helping relationships.

In sum, the experts have failed the public, but who will be held accountable? Perhaps the entire edifice of psychopharmacotherapy must be dismantled and rebuilt from scratch. In such a renewed and more democratic endeavor, participation from *anyone* who wishes to participate should be welcomed as long as their contributions—which cannot, in this interest-conflicted mental health field, be guaranteed to be principled—are transparent.

REFERENCES

Antonuccio, D. O., Danton, W. G., & McClanahan, T. M. (2003). Psychology in the prescription era: Building a firewall between marketing and science. *American Psychologist, 58,* 1028–1043.

Armstrong, D., & Mathews, A. W. (2004, May 14). Pfizer case signals tougher action on off–label drug use. *Wall Street Journal,* p. B1.

Austrian, S. G. (2000). *Mental disorders, medications, and clinical social work* (2nd edition). New York: Columbia University Press.

Bentley, K. J. (2003). (Ed.). Psychiatric medication issues for social workers, counselors, and psychologists [Special Issue]. *Social Work in Mental Health, 1*(4).

Bentley, K. J., & Walsh, J. (2001). *The social worker and psychotropic medication: Toward effective collaboration between mental health clients, families, and providers* (2nd edition). Boston: Wadsworth Publishing.

Bentley, K. J., Walsh, J., & Farmer, R. (2005). Referring clients for psychiatric medication: Best practices for social workers. *Best Practices in Mental Health, 1*(1), 59–71.

Braslow, J. (1997). *Mental ills and bodily cures: Psychiatric treatment in the first half of the twentieth century.* Berkeley: University of California Press.

Breggin, P.R., & Cohen, D. (1999). *Your drug may be your problem: How and why to stop taking psychiatric medications.* Cambridge, MA: Perseus.

Cauchon, D. (2000, September 25). FDA advisors tied to industry. *USA Today,* pp. 1A, 10A.

Chalmers, I. (1990). Underreporting research is scientific misconduct. *JAMA, 263,* 1405–1408.

Cohen, D. (1997a). A critique of the use of neuroleptic drugs in psychiatry. In S. Fisher & R. G. Greenberg (Eds.), *From placebo to panacea: Putting psychiatric drugs to the test* (pp. 173–228). New York: Wiley.

Cohen, D. (1997b). Psychiatrogenics: Introducing chlorpromazine in psychiatry. *Review of Existential Psychology and Psychiatry, 23* (1–2), 206–233.

Cohen, D. (2003). The psychiatric medication history: Context, purpose, and method. *Social Work in Mental Health, 4,* 5–28.

Cohen, D. (2005). Clinical psychopharmacology trials: "Gold standard" or "fool's gold"? In S. Kirk (ed.), *Mental disorders in the social environment: Perspectives from social work* (pp. 347–367). New York: Columbia University Press.

Cohen, D., & Karsenty, S. (1998). *Représentations sociales des effets secondaires des anxiolytiques: Une étude comparative Québec-France.* [Social representations of the side effects of anxiolytic drugs: A comparative Quebec-France study]. Research report submitted to Ministry of Health & Municipal Affairs, France.

Cohen, D., McCubbin, M., Collin, J., & Perodeau, G. (2001). Medications as social phenomena. *Health, 5,* 441–469.

Conrad, P., & Schneider, J. (1992). *Deviance and medicalization: From badness to sickness* (2nd ed.). Philadelphia, PA: Temple University Press.

Depressing research. (2004). *Lancet, 363*, 1335.

Diekelmann, N. L., & Kavanagh, K H. (Eds.). (2002). *First, do no harm: Power, oppression, and violence in healthcare*. Madison, WI: University of Wisconsin Press.

Dolnick, E. (1998). *Madness on the couch: Blaming the victim in the heyday of psychoanalysis*. New York: Simon & Schuster.

Dziegielewski, S. F., & Leon, A. M. (2001). *Social work practice and psychopharmacology*. New York: Springer Publishing Company.

Fancher, R. (1995). *Cultures of healing: Correcting the image of American mental health care*. San Francisco: Freeman.

Farmer, R., & Bentley, K. J. (2002). Social workers as medication facilitators. In K. J. Bentley (Ed.), *Social work practice in mental health: Contemporary roles, tasks, and techniques* (pp. 211–229). Pacific Grove, CA: Brooks/Cole.

Fava, (2004). Conflict of interest in psychopharmacology: Can Dr. Jekyll still control Mr. Hyde? *Psychotherapy & Psychosomatics, 73*, 1–4.

Floersch, J. (2002). *Meds, money, and manners: The case management of severe mental illness*. New York: Columbia University Press.

Fortune. (2000). How the industries stack up. Available from http://money.cnn.com/ magazines/fortune_archive/2000/04/17/278092/index.htm

Fukuyama, F. (2002). *Our posthuman future: Consequences of the biotechnology revolution*. New York: Farrar, Straus, and Giroux.

Gibbs, L., & Gambrill, E. (1999). *Critical thinking for social workers: Exercises for the helping professions*. Thousand Oaks, CA: Pine Forge Press.

Grinspoon, L., & Hedblom, P. (1975). *The speed culture: Amphetamine use and abuse in America*. Cambridge, MA: Harvard University Press.

Harris, G. (2003, August 7). Debate resumes over the safety of depression's wonder drugs. *New York Times*, p. A1.

Harris, G. (2004a, June 3). Spitzer sues a drug maker, saying it hid negative data. *New York Times*, pp. A1, C4.

Harris, G. (2004b, April 16). Expert kept from speaking at antidepressant hearing. *New York Times*, p. A–16.

Healy, D. (1997). *The antidepressant era*. New York: Harvard University Press.

Healy, D. (2002). *The creation of psychopharmacology*. New York: Harvard University Press.

Hegarty, J. D., Baldessarini, R. J., Tohen, M., Waternaux, C., & Oepen, G. (1994). One hundred years of schizophrenia: A meta-analysis of the outcome literature. *American Journal of Psychiatry, 151*, 1409–1416.

Hoehn-Saric, R., Lipsey, J. R., & McLeod, D. A. (1990). Apathy and indifference in patients on fluvoxamine and fluoxetine. *Journal of Clinical Psychopharmacology, 10*, 343–345.

Horton, R. (2004). The dawn of Mcscience. *New York Review of Books*, 51(4). Retrieved April 4, 2004 from http://www.nybooks.com/articles

Illich, I. (1976). *Limits to medicine. Medical nemesis: The expropriation of health*. Toronto: McClelland and Stewart Limited.

IMS Health. (2003, February 28). 2002 world pharma sales growth: Slower, but still healthy. Retrieved June 16, 2003 from http://www.ims-global.com/insight/news_story/0302/news_story_030228.htm

Jacobs, D., & Cohen, D. (1999). What is really known about psychological alterations produced by psychiatric drugs? *International Journal of Risk and Safety in Medicine, 12,* 37–47.

Judge: Paxil ads "misleading." (2002, August 21). *CBS News.* Retrieved April 15, 2004 from http://www.cbsnews.com/stories/2002/08/20/health/main519266.shtml

Johnson, A. B. (1990). *Out of Bedlam: The truth about deinstitutionalization.* New York: Basic Books.

Johnson, L. A. (2004, May 17). Behavior drug spending eclipses other youth meds. *The Standard Times.* Retrieved May 17, 2004 from http://www.southcoasttoday.com/daily/05-04/05-17-04/a05wn.htm

Jureidini, J. N., Doecke, C. J., Mansfield, P.R., Haby, M.M., Menkes, D. B., & Tonkin, A.L. (2004). Efficacy and safety of antidepressants for children and adolescents. *British Medical Journal, 328,* 879–883.

Kessler, R. A., Berglund, P., Demler, O., Jin, R., Koretz, D., Merikanga, K. R., Rush, A. J., Walters, E. E., & Wang, P. S. (2003). The epidemiology of major depressive disorder: Results from the National Comorbidity Survey Replication. *JAMA, 289,* 3095–3105.

Kirsch, I., Moore, T. J., Scoboria, A., & Nicholls, S.N. (2002). The Emperor's new drugs: An analysis of antidepressant medication data submitted to the U.S. Food and Drug Administration. *Prevention & Treatment, 5,* article 23. Available at http://journals.apa.org/prevention/volume5/toc-jul15-02.htm

Kondro W., & Sibbald, B. (2004). Drug company experts advised staff to withhold data about SSRI use in children: A 1993–1996 industry study showed that paroxetine was no more effective than placebo in treating pediatric depression. *Canadian Medical Association Journal, 170,* 783.

Kranish, M. (2002, December 22). FDA counsel's rise embodies US shift. *Boston Globe.* Retrieved April 16 2004 from http://www.bostonglobe.com

Lacasse, J.F., & Gomory, T. (2003). Is graduate social work education promoting a critical approach to mental health practice? *Journal of Social Work Education, 39,* 383–408.

Meier, B. (2004, June 21). A medical journal quandary: Jow to report on drug trials. *New York Times,* p. A–1.

Medawar, C., & Hardon, A. (2004). *Medicines out of control? Antidepressants and the conspiracy of goodwill.* London: Aksant Academic Publishers/Transaction.

Mental health: A report from the Surgeon General. (1999). Washington: Office of the Surgeon General.

Mirowsky, J., & Ross, C. E. (2003). *Social causes of psychological distress* (2nd ed.). Chicago: Aldine de Gruyter.

Moncrieff, J., & Cohen, D. (2005). Rethinking models of psychotropic drug action. *Psychotherapy & Psychosomatics, 73,* 145–153.

Morgan, R.F. (Ed.). (1983). *The iatrogenics handbook: A critical look at research and practice in the helping professions.* Toronto: IPI Publishing.

National Center for Health Statistics. (2005). *Health United States, 2004.* Retrieved February 15, 2005 from http://www.cdc.gov/nchs/hus.htm

Nesse, R. M., & Berridge, K. C. (1997). Psychoactive drug use in evolutionary perspective. *Science, 278*(5335), 63–66.

New 2001 data shows big drug companies spent almost two-and-one-half times as much on marketing, advertising, and administration as they spent on research and development. (2002). FamiliesUSA. Retrieved June 5, 2004 from: http://www.familiesusa.org/site/PageServer?pagename=new2001data

Patten, S. B. (2004). The impact of population treatment on population health: Synthesis of data from two national sources in Canada. *Population Health Metrics, 2*(9). Available online: http://www.pophealthmetrics.com/content/2/1/9

Peterson, (2004, February 1). Making drugs, shaping the rules. *New York Times*, p. A1.

Procyshin, R. M., Chan, A., Fortin, P., & Jenkins, W. (2004). Prevalence and outcome of pharmaceutical industry – sponsored clinical trials involving clozapine, risperidone, or olanzapine. *Canadian Journal of Psychiatry, 49*(9), 601–606.

Relman, A. S., & Angell, M. (2002, December 16). America's other drug problem: How the drug industry disorts medicine and politics. *The New Republic*, pp. 27–41.

Research Triangle Institute. (2002). *Screening for depression: Systematic evidence review.* Rockville, MD: Agency for Health Care Quality and Research.

Sharav, V. H. (2004). Conflicts of interests policy-New York Times. *Alliance for Human Research Protection.* Available at: http://www.ahrp.org/infomail/04/03/28.html

Sharav, V. H. (2003). Children in clinical research: A conflict of moral values. *American Journal of Bioethics, InFocus*, pp. 1–81. Retrieved May 7, 2003 from http://bioethics.net

Shogren, E. (2004). FDA sat on report linking suicide, drugs. *Los Angeles Times.* Retrieved April 6, 2004 from http://www.latimes.com/news/nationworld/nation/la-na-suicide6apr06,1,2908070.story?coll=la-headlines-nation

Smith, D. C. (2001). On the incompatibility of the biological and empathic-relational model. *Ethical Human Sciences and Services, 3*, 47–52.

Smith, R. (2005). Medical journals are an extension of the marketing arm of pharmaceutical companies, *PLoS Medicine, 2*(5), e138.

Sullivan, R. J., & Hagen, E. H. (2002). Psychotropic substance-seeking: Evolutionary pathology or adaptation? *Addiction, 97*, 389–400.

Szasz, T. (1974). *Ceremonial chemistry: The ritual persecution of drugs, addicts, and pushers.* New York: Anchor Press/Doubleday.

Van Praag, H. M. (2002). Why has the antidepressant era not shown a significant drop in suicide rates? *Crisis, 23*, 77–82.

Vastag, B. (2001). Pay attention: Ritalin acts much like cocaine. *JAMA, 286*, 905–906.

Wagner, K. D., Robb, A. S., Findling, R. L., Jin, J., Gutierrez, M. M., & Heydorn, W. E. (2004). A randomized, placebo-controlled trial of citalopram for the treatment of major depression in children and adolescents. *American Journal of Psychiatry, 161*, 1079–1083.

Walsh, J., Farmer, R., Taylor, M., & Bentley, K. J. (2003). Ethical dilemmas of practicing social workers around psychiatric medication: Results of a national study. *Social Work in Mental health, 1*(4), 91–105.

Waters, R. (2004, April 16). FDA was urged to limit kids' antidepressants. Advice citing risk of suicide rejected. *San Francisco Chronicle*, p. A–1.

Whitaker, R. (2002). *Mad in America: Bad science, bad medicine, and the enduring mistreatment of the mentally ill.* Cambridge, MA: Perseus.

Whittington, C. J., Kendall, T., Fonagy, P., Cottrell, D., Cotgrove, A., & Boddington, E. (2004). Selective serotonin reuptake inhibitors in childhood depression: Systematic review of published versus unpublished data. *The Lancet, 363*, 1341–1345.

Wilman, D. (2004, April 9). Curbs on outside deals at NIH urged. *Los Angeles Times.* Retrieved April 15, 2004 from http://latimes.com/la-na-nihapr09,1,1273370.story

Beyond Survivorship: Achieving a Harmonious Dynamic Equilibrium Using a Chinese Medicine Framework in Health and Mental Health

S. M. Ng, PhD
Cecilia L. W. Chan, PhD
Pamela P. Y. Leung, PhD
Celia H. Y. Chan, MSW, RSW
Josephine K. Y. Yau, MPhil, MSSc

CHINESE MEDICINE—FACILITATING SELF-HEALING THROUGH REBALANCING THE SYSTEM

Social work in health care is heavily influenced by Western medicine that focuses on illness, disease, germs, malfunctions, and disabilities.[1] Molecular and genetic investigation of the brain, however, can neither fully explain depression nor provide an adequate solution for life-style-related problems. Recent trends in search of alternative solutions to health and well-being from a total person perspective have laid the platform for health care professionals and social workers to look for guidance from traditional wisdom. Very few traditional medicines survive since Western medicine has prevailed. Chinese medicine is one of them (WHO, 2002). It survives not because Chinese herbs are especially potent. It is the unique philosophical and theoretical sophistication of Chinese medicine that brings our understanding of health and illness to new heights (Ng, 2003).

The fundamental theoretical framework of Chinese medicine was established over 2000 years ago. The Inner Canon of Medicine, written in the 1st Century BC, laid the basic foundation for the development of Chinese medicine (Wang, Chiu, & Hong, 2000). Two core theories characterize Chinese medicine: the holistic perspective, and syndromatic diagnosis as the basis of treatment formulation (Cai, 1995). In a nutshell, Chinese medicine emphasizes total well-being by facilitating the self-healing of the individual through rebalancing their intrapersonal and interpersonal systems. The person's mind-body-spiritual systems and the person in relation to the environment are all crucial in the maintenance of good health.

Holistic Perspective

Chinese medicine adopts a dynamic, systemic perspective in understanding the functioning of a person. The body is made up of various internal organ systems that are tightly connected by a comprehensive network of meridians. At the same time, the mind is another complex system that comprises cognitions, emotions, values, morality, and beliefs. Being tightly connected and intensively interacting with each other, mind and body together form a holistic higher-level system. Chinese medicine's holistic perspective actually goes beyond the body. It is also concerned about the relationship between the person and the social and natural world. Deriving harmony within the body and the mind, as well as between the self and the environment, form the basis for good health.

Syndromatic Diagnosis as the Basis of Treatment Formulation

In Chinese medicine, there are two levels of diagnosis: disease diagnosis and syndromatic diagnosis (Li & Yang, 1999). Disease diagnosis is conceptually the same as that in Western medicine, though the two systems have their own disease classification system. Syndromatic diagnosis is something unique to Chinese medicine. It is a diagnosis of disequilibrium among the subsystems. Chinese medicine strongly advocates that restoring an equilibrium can help the organism heal itself. It is an orientation toward the facilitation of self-healing. Such intervention is regarded as fundamental.

In Chinese medicine, neither the disease agents nor the symptoms are the key targets of treatment. The primary treatment target is the system imbalance, and therefore the treatment focuses on restoring the harmonious dynamic equilibrium among various body and mind subsystems. In clinical practice, this approach works very well in many diseases, including conditions that Western medicine can do very little about. For example, Chinese medicine is known for its treatment of viral infections without using any antivirus herbs but by strengthening immunity. Chinese medicine also works well in many functional disorders, such as irritable bowel syndrome, which is highly prevalent and with a multifactorial etiology (Bensoussan & Talley, 1998).

Treatments in Chinese medicine are not limited to physical treatments like herbal medicine and acupuncture. Chinese medicine favors a multimodal intervention approach that includes nutritional therapy, traditional health exercises like Tai Chi and Qigong, counseling, and a quest for spirituality based on traditional Chinese philosophies, like Confucianism, Daoism, and Buddhism. Great flexibility and creativity are allowed in tailor-making a treatment plan for a client. The baseline is that the treatment combination must be formulated in line with the holistic thinking and aim at rebalancing the overall system.

This strengthening, non-antagonistic, and holistic treatment approach is the core treatment philosophy of Chinese medicine. It also sheds new light on psychosocial intervention. This article will discuss how the holistic Chinese Medicine framework of facilitating self-healing through rebalancing the system and achieving a harmonious dynamic equilibrium can be used in psychosocial intervention.

EXAMPLE OF EMOTIONAL HEALING FROM THE CHINESE MEDICINE PERSPECTIVE—EXCESSIVE ANGER

Chinese medicine sees all emotions—anger, joy, worry, sorrow, fear, etc.—as normal and essential to well-being. It does not classify them into positive and negative emotions. Instead, it believes that to be truly alive, one needs to fully experience all emotions. The key point is to maintain an appropriate dynamic equilibrium among them.

Problems arise when an emotion is either stagnated or excessive. This triggers an imbalance in the system. For example, excessive anger can lead to a series of changes in other emotions. With reference to the Five Elements Theory,[2] anger facilitates joy and represses worry (Chan, Ho, & Chow,

2001). Therefore, excessive anger leads to excessive joy and deficient worry. The person can go into a manic state with high impulsivity. When anger is totally blocked off, the person has no motivation to live and can easily move into a depression or panic attack. The ripple effect can go on as joy and worry affect other emotions. In a nutshell, the dynamic equilibrium of the system is upset. The clinical presentation is that the person exhibits excessive anger, which is intermittently replaced by excessive joy. The rapid switching between the two emotions can be very dramatic. Because of reduced worry, the person can be impulsive in decision making and behavior. Pachuta (1989, p. 84–85) wrote:

> *Anger is mothered by fear and controlled by grief. Hence whenever you are angry, it would be useful to ask, "What am I afraid of? What am I sad about?" . . . Since anger is generated by fear, it follows that the most violent anger is indicative of the greatest fear . . . The emotion under guilt is fear, the fear of retribution . . . Fear is controlled by empathy . . . The antidote for grief is love and joy. Joy is the major preventer and cure of depression . . . Anger is the antidote for sympathy . . . Grief is the antidote for and controller of anger.*

To rectify the imbalance, there are several options: reducing fear (which will therefore become less facilitative on anger), increasing sorrow (which will therefore become more repressive on anger), and reducing joy (which will therefore become less repressive on sorrow which will in turn become more repressive on anger). Hence, there are multiple entry points for intervention. In ancient times, Chinese medicine practitioners could be very directive in manipulating these emotions. Applying such concepts nowadays in mental health practice, we adopt a more psychoeducational and facilitative stance. We facilitate the exploration of various emotions. The objective is to remove blockage so that the system will regain the necessary fluidity and rebalance itself.

Because of the mind-body connection, excessive anger will hurt the liver system. According to the meridian theory and Chinese Medicine observations, excessive liver *qi* (energy) will travel up along the sides of the chest (often leading to side chest pain) to the eyes (often leading to reddish eyes) and the brain (often leading to emotional and sleep disturbance). According to the Five Elements Theory, an excessive liver system is repressive of the spleen (digestive) system, resulting in gastrointestinal symptoms. Hence, physical treatments of excessive anger will often include the "softening of the liver system" and the "strengthening of the spleen (digestive) system." The underpinning treatment philosophy is to rebalance the system. That can be achieved through herbal medicine, acupuncture, and nutritional therapy. Nonphysical means, like traditional health exercises, counseling, massage, acupressure, and pursuing spirituality are also employed. A multimodal intervention approach is believed to be most effective in fostering holistic well-being.

Use of the Chinese Medicine Framework in Psychosocial Intervention

Strongly influenced by mind-body dualistic thinking and the scientific paradigm of reductionism, Western medicine and cultures perceive different human domains as discrete entities (Abramson, 2003; Chan, et al., 2001; Engel, 1977). This dualistic and reductionist thinking limits itself in accessing and utilizing the potential of the different healing capacities of human beings. The development of psychotherapy also reflects this compartmentalized trend. For instance, psychoanalysis focuses on intrapsychic forces, while behaviorism emphasizes observable behavior. They put primacy on one domain of human experience while downplaying the others (Chan et al., 2001).

The development of mind-body medicine, the biopsychosocial health model, and the increasing recognition of the power of the mind and body process suggested by hypnosis, biofeedback, psychosomatic phenomena, and mindfulness practice represent the increasing recognition of the field in reconnecting the mind and the body (Engel, 1977; Ogden, 2000). There is a growing interest in how the Chinese medicine framework can shed light on clinical practice in health and mental health (Chan et al., 2001; Wong & McKeen, 1998). Inspired by the Chinese medical perspective, the authors developed a body-mind-spirit model of intervention in health and mental health. This model stresses that body, mind, and spirit are an integrated whole. All problems physical or mental, are at their root related to imbalances in the multilayered system. Striving to regain balance and harmony both within the person and between the person and the environment becomes the fundamental goal in healing. This is achieved through a process of change that builds on the self-healing capacities of individuals. Such a concept necessitates a revisiting of assumptions, therapy goals, and the therapeutic process underlying this model.

Assumptions and Therapy Goals of the Body-Mind-Spirit Model

There are a number of assumptions behind this model.

1. Everything is connected. Human existence is a manifestation of physical, emotional, cognitive, social, and spiritual being. The different domains are interconnected and come together to form a whole. Human existence is also connected to the social, interpersonal environment and the wider universe.
2. Life is the eternal dance of Yin and Yang. Life is ever changing. Energy flows in creating a harmonious dynamic equilibrium. Problems in living, including ill health, are caused by disruption to the balance of Yin and Yang energies.
3. Healing comes from within. Therapy aims to ignite the person's own healing power and to bring the person back into a state of balance. Intervention looks for strengths rather than pathologies.
4. Restoring harmony not only cures illness and resolves problems, but it also opens up opportunities for growth and transformation.

This model represents a different approach than that of Western mainstream therapy. Instead of perceiving human domains as discrete entities, it views them as interconnected. While Western interventions are largely problem-oriented and focus on removing symptoms for restoring health and well-being, our approach goes beyond symptom removal and survivorship. Symptom reduction that focuses on emancipating an individual from problems represents only one end of the continuum of therapy goals. Personal growth and transformation represents the other end of that continuum. Body-mind-spirit intervention aims for transformation and the attainment of harmonious dynamic equilibrium within the self, with others, and with the universe.

A person who goes through a crisis may experience a disruption in one or more of the body, mind, and spiritual domains. The goal of intervention is to induce changes in the tripartite system to regain a new balance. Our goal is not only to help a person to survive a crisis, but to go beyond it. We believe that people are not only able to bounce back to the pre-crisis functioning level, but can exceed it by using the crisis experience as a springboard to further individual growth. We aim to achieve a new balance in which a person is revitalized. The person is not only able to endure pain, but also able to see the gain that goes with the pain. A balanced person realizes that suffering may not be eradicated, and that it can co-exist with a sense of peace, contentment, and tranquility. Suffering becomes an impetus for one to turn crises into opportunities. One is able to exhibit inner strength and to realize latent human potentiality.

This concept is echoed by the increasing popularity of positive psychology (Seligman & Csikszentmihalyi, 2000) and health psychology (Friedman, 2002; Ogden, 2000) in recent years. People surviving trauma, growing, and becoming more resilient are widely reported in recent studies (Bonanno, 2004; Park, 1998; Tedeschi & Calhoun, 1996). Recent studies in both Western and Eastern populations also confirm that enhancing positive coping and positive emotions rather than reducing negative coping and negative emotions facilitates growth and well-being (Ho, Chan, & Ho, 2004; Huppert & Whittington, 2003). Inspired by the Chinese medicine perspective, the body-mind-spirit model primarily aims at igniting the person's own strength and healing power by bringing that person back into a state of dynamic equilibrium.

The Harmonization Process

The Body-Mind-Spirit approach involves mobilizing the interconnected parts through a multimodal intervention approach—working on the body, mind and spiritual domains. It involves a harmonization process in four stages.

Stage One—Awareness of Disharmony and Imbalance of the System: The traumatic event leads to disintegration at multiple levels—between body and mind, various internal systems within the self, between the self and others, and between the self and the environemt. Intervention at this stage focuses on facilitating genuine acknowledgement and acceptance of losses. Failure to acknowledge losses results in the stagnation of energy flow, which may result in bodily or psychological symptom manifestations.

Stage Two—Strengthening the System to Restore Balance: Intervention focuses on enhancing internal physical and mental strength to attain harmony, strengthening the vital *qi* (energy flow) and the body's self-healing ability to ensure that the positive changes are sustainable.

Stage Three—Harmonization of Body and Mind: Interventions focus on facilitating recognition of the interconnectedness of body and mind, acceptance, letting go, and living in the present moment with a peace of mind.

Stage Four—Spiritual Transformation: This involves revitalizing life energy to attain a grounded self that is fully connected with others, nature, the universe or higher power. While a goal-oriented pathway of life is redefined, the course of life is also fully appreciated and experienced. This is achieved through deriving new meaning in life and reconstructing spirituality. A shift away from being overly self-focused is often useful at this stage. An effective strategy is to encourage the development of dedication in helping others. Human potential is maximized through transformation.

Throughout these stages of harmonization, the goal of intervention is to stimulate the body's own self-healing abilities and to facilitate an undisturbed flow of energy within the body-mind-spirit interconnected web. Body-mind-spirit harmony is the foundation for living fully. In a disharmonized state, extreme dissipation of energy may lead to various psychopathological states. If the energy is turned inwards, there can be depression, self harm, and guilt. If the energy is turned outwards, there can be conflict, violence, and destruction. In a harmonized state, energy flows smoothly in a dynamic equilibrium. The following section will describe the process in more detail and discuss the techniques involved.

Connecting and Strengthening the Body

Our body has the natural ability to maintain a steady state in our body processes and with the external environment, that is, to maintain an equilibrium (Green & Shellenberger, 1991). However, while the body is trying to attain harmony in one part, it may create imbalance in another. For example, Chinese people, under the influence of Confucian teaching on social harmony, may sacrifice their own well-being for the fulfillment of collective well-being. In such a case, the person is in harmony with the bigger social system while compromising his/her own physical and psychological well-being. The somatization of psychosocial problems is common among the Chinese people. It is helpful to use the body as an entry point in the therapeutic process where the client can get connected with their self and be aware of the interconnectedness of the body and the mind. At the beginning of the harmonization process, our focus is on the awareness of disharmony and on strengthening the system. Techniques for connecting and nurturing the body include: body scanning to identify energy stagnation points, breathing, therapeutic massage, Tai Chi and Qigong exercise to facilitate the flow of *qi* (life energy), psycho-education on food and tonics, and the development of a healthy lifestyle.

Awareness of energy stagnation through body scanning: As human beings are integrated wholes, any problem in either the mind or the spirit domain will also affect the body. Connecting with a client by listening to their physical pain and discomfort is usually a good entry point. Body scanning is a simple and fast-engaging technique that helps people to get in touch with their bodies. Clients are helped to go into a relaxing but mindful state. They are taught to consciously focus attention on their body and attempt not to be distracted by ruminations. They are then instructed to focus attention on their different body parts. By scanning through their whole body, they become aware of the parts that experience pain or discomfort. These are usually where energy flow is blocked or stagnated. In the very process of getting in touch with the body and being aware of any energy stagnation, one may also become connected with one's own mind and spirit, as energy stagnation in the body is usually mirrored by fixation in our mind (Wong & McKeen, 1998). According to the five elements theory of Chinese medicine, complaints about different bodily organs reflect different forms of emotional disharmony. For example, an extremely angry person usually has a problem related to the liver and gall bladder system; lung system problems are associated with excess sorrow; those who worry or contemplate too much are likely to experience problems related to the digestive system (Chan et al., 2001; Yin et al., 1994). These explanations may not fit everyone perfectly because of individual differences. However, they provide quick entry points for connecting with the client, and help the client to connecting their own mind and body. This also highlights the importance of achieving mind-body harmony as a therapeutic goal.

Facilitating the flow of *qi* (life energy): There is a Chinese belief that life energy (*qi*) flows through the meridians of our bodies. Breathing can be used as a powerful tool to facilitate the flow of the *qi*. It can also restore stability of the body and mind when we are mindful of our breathing. Mindful breathing helps us be in touch with our deep emotion, whether it is pain, fear, anger, joy, or contentment. Breathing changes with our moods, and vice versa. It can be used to harmonize our mood as it helps regulate the flow of *qi* and vitalize it. In deep breathing, one enters a state of total concentration and consciousness. People in a state of supreme consciousness are able to connect with the others and the universe as well as obtain a deeper understanding of their own spiritual existence. We always teach our clients simple breathing meditation techniques. Sometimes, suggestions are given to invite them to breathe in the vital energy from the nurturing universe and breathe out the negative energy from the body. In more advanced practice, we suggest that patients breathe out compassionate loving energy, care, and concern to people around them. Clients say that breathing helps them to refresh their minds and become more grounded.

> *Ms. Lee had been suffering from mood and sleep disturbance since she was diagnosed as having breast cancer a year before. She practiced breathing meditation for 15 minutes before bedtime every day. Because of weakness in her legs, she did not adopt the lotus sitting position, which is preferred in meditation. Instead, she simply sat on a chair with her back as straight and upright as possible. The practice included an imagery component—breathing in vital energy and breathing out negative emotions. When the mindful state was interrupted by "automatic thinking," she was taught not to confront the thinking. She simply took note of it and then gently brought her attention back to the breathing. After about one week of regular practice, the sleep problem disappeared and Ms. Lee's mood improved. She said that in meditation she became aware of her internal emotions and got connected with them. Energy previously got stuck started to flow again, as manifested by a revitalized body. The result was a better mind-body balance.*

Therapeutic massage: Chinese medicine uses acupuncture and acupressure to stimulate the meridians of our body, regulate the flow of *qi*, restore its healthy circulation, and enhance immune functioning (Beinfield & Korngold, 2003). In the context of psychosocial intervention, simple light acupressure and massage are fun, easy to learn, and safe. More importantly, they bring a lot of energy to the therapeutic process. Prescribing therapeutic massage to couples or parents and children helps enhance marital or family relationships. Massaging one another is a powerful way of expressing concern and love; sometimes it works better than words. Based on knowledge of traditional Chinese medicine, we developed and packaged the practice of acupressure, therapeutic massage, and breathing techniques as simple and easy-to-learn "one-second techniques" that can be readily incorporated in a counseling session (Chan, 2001).

Tai Chi and Qigong exercises: Tai Chi and Qigong are forms of mind-body exercise characterized by slowness in movement (Hung, 1993). The slowness is deliberate and serves two purposes. First, it helps to train the inner strength and endurance of the body. Second, it demands total concentration in the mind and a high degree of awareness of the bodily movement. As a result, it facilitates mind-body connection and harmony.

Madam Yu had been suffering from ruminations of ungrounded worries about her children's academic performance for about ten years. She had tried a number of cognitive and behavioral techniques to stop the ruminations, but they were in vain. A month ago, she started attending a Tai Chi class every morning. She happily reported that she was in a state of tranquility when practicing Tai Chi. She had missed such mind-body harmony for a long time. Although such a state could not be maintained for the rest of the day, the wonderful experience of a balanced state was already encouraging enough to boost her confidence in further tackling her ruminations.

Psycho-education on food, tonics, and diet: Many people in distress neglect taking good care of their body and do not have good diets. Because of the mind-body interconnectedness, a vicious cycle can easily be set off. This can be found in many of our clients. To stop the vicious cycle, one needs to correct the diet and lifestyle habits. First we need to pay attention to the quality, quantity, and frequency of the food intake. According to Chinese medicine, the diet needs to be constantly adjusted in view of individual differences, their health and physical conditions of the time (Ng, 2003). In our therapeutic sessions, we teach our clients to design the most suitable diet by constantly listening to their bodies and getting in touch with the changing environment. It is a ritual to be able to love our body and respect nature.

Healthy lifestyle: In face of distress, many people adopt maladaptive behavior in the hope of escaping from the discomfort. Some examples of such behavior are indulgence in certain material comforts, eating, shopping, gambling, smoking, drinking, sexual pleasure, and speed driving. These strategies can only at best offer a temporary relief. The distress remains and, very often, becomes even worse because of the indulgence in high-risk behavior. Influenced by Daoism, Chinese medicine advocates a simple life, contained desires, and respect for nature. In our therapeutic sessions, we show our clients how to achieve harmony with their desires and with nature. To fully enjoy and appreciate life, we can pay attention to what we have instead of what we do not have. A sense of contentment can greatly enhance mind-body-spirit harmony.

Mr. Fong sought temporary haven by seeking sexual pleasure at nightclubs. Very quickly, he had to go to nightclubs at least three times a week. The therapist helped Mr. Fong to explore the consequences of continued indulgence in his body. He was motivated to change and reverted to a simple life. He gained a more harmonized mind-body state in about two weeks time. The newly gained harmony provided a foundation for further therapeutic work.

Harmonizing the Mind and Body

There is only one Chinese word for "mind" and "heart": "*Xin*". *Xin* is a complex construct that encompasses the physical heart, a sound mind, passion, care, concern, will power, vision, hope, emotion, reflection, carefulness, human sensitivity, and cognition. *Xin* denotes physique, personality, values, and emotions. Harmonizing the mind involves a 3-A process: acknowledging vulnerability, accepting the adversity and unpredictability of life, and activating one's self-healing capacity.

Acknowledging vulnerability: Influenced by Buddhist teaching, we help patients to normalize their suffering as a part of life. Old age, sickness, and death are the natural course in life, and the related sufferings are just part of the law of nature. By acknowledging our own vulnerability and normalizing suffering, we can face pain and losses with a tranquil mind.

Accepting adversity and unpredictability of life: Acceptance is different from resignation. Resignation represents a state of assuming a victim role, whereas acceptance involves the peaceful understanding of the reality of the situation. "*Acceptance is not a passive surrendering, but rather an act of taking responsibility; it is not blaming oneself for having the disease, but working energetically to restore one's system to balance.*" (Abramson, 2003, p. 20). Acceptance means fully embracing whatever is in the present. People who embrace losses are more ready to appreciate gains through suffering. As Lao-zi, the founder of Daoism, described, "*It is suffering that gives way to bliss; it is in bliss that suffering reveals.*" (*Lao-zi*, 6th century B.C.) Balance and harmony imply the ability to appreciate gains and losses as an intermingled essence of everyday living. Crisis creates imbalance in life, but the opportunity that goes with the crisis will bring about a new balance in life.

Activating the self-healing capacity: The key to activating the capacity for self-healing is to let go. By letting go of intense emotional attachment, we can free our energy for self-healing. Buddhism teaches people not to cling to things or persons, as attachment and desire are sources of suffering. Emotional attachment and holding on to desire are the roots of many forms of energy stagnation and disharmony. While Western forms of therapy largely work to help patients better master, control, and overcome the problems at hand, Buddhist teaching encourages an individual to detach and to let go so that they can flow with moment by moment experiences instead of being controlled by or preoccupied with desires. Paradoxically, one gains control by letting go of control. By practicing emotional detachment and letting go, people find it easier to forgive. Letting go and genuine forgiveness are the ultimate solutions to all emotional problems. They free people from enmeshed relationships and disturbed emotions that are caused by interpersonal attachment. They also resolve frustration that is caused by unmet expectations. Balance in energy flow and internal well-being is regained. In our experience of working with Chinese cancer patients, bereaved widows, and divorced women, we found clients' self-healing power largely ignited from the determination in letting go of the victim role and starting a new life. In the counseling sessions, we often invite our clients to read affirmation statements like "I am determine to let go of the past and to live a new life", "I choose to love myself" and "I am the Master of my own life" aloud. If individuals can free themselves from sick patterns and discover more of their inner self, they can regain a state of well-being (Wong & McKeen, 1998).

> *Mrs. Lee was feeling very insecure because life could be vulnerable and unpredictable. She worried that her oldest son was taking the risk of starting a venture business while he was only an undergraduate student. She worried that her son indulged too much in dating and did not exert enough effort in his studies. She worried that he would eventually be expelled from the university. She worried that her son's failure in university studies would be known to her neighbors . . . She was living in constant worry and became very sick mentally and physically. Consciously or unconsciously, she was using her sick role to win back control over her son. That was a battle with no winners. Every family member was sucked into it and suffered immensely. In the counseling process, Mrs. Lee was helped to see that paving a "safe path" for her son was an illusion. The world was unpredictable. True safety was about peace of mind and not about controlling the path to the future. Accepting unpredictability was the first step. The second step was letting go of the desire to control through being sick or playing the victim role. She was enlightened and changed dramatically to become a relaxed and happy mother.*

Other techniques of mobilizing the power of the mind include meditation, guided imagery, and mindfulness exercises. According to Collins Gem English Learner's Dictionary, the word "meditate" means "think seriously about something." The emphasis is on thinking. In Eastern meditation practice, however, the emphasis is just the opposite—not thinking. Meditation is about freeing oneself from the dominance of thinking to achieve a conscious state of holistic being. If the person is fixated in cognitive preoccupation, meditation techniques that help one become mindful of their total existence in the present moment can free the fixed energy and allow it to move in a more fluid manner. Harmonious balance can be regained. Some meditation practices can be very elaborate and complicated. In psychosocial intervention, we avoid religion-specific rituals and just focus on achieving the core objective—mindfulness. There is a growing body of evidence that supports the mental health benefits of mindfulness training (Baer, 2003). In our sessions, we teach and facilitate simple breathing meditation, mindful eating, tea-drinking, and body movements. Sometimes, we add guided imagery in the course of meditation. The imagery may be a mental haven for fostering peace and tranquility. It may also be used for fostering loving-kindness and forgiveness.

Spiritual Transformation and Harmonization

Spiritual transformation is the ultimate goal of our harmonizing intervention. This involves a process of reorganizing and revitalizing oneself to a new fluid, balanced state of total being. The transformed client is not only able to endure pain peacefully, but is also able to live life more fully, and has a re-organized and integrated goal-oriented life. In our clinical experience, many of the transformed clients shift away from an overly self-focused life to being dedicated to helping others. Meaning reconstruction and appreciation are key components in this stage.

Meaning Reconstruction: To make sense of the world and the happenings in life, people develop a schema that sets out some fundamental assumptions about the world and the self. These worldviews and views about the self are relatively stable. People generally feel comfortable if these views are in harmony with their appraisal of events that they have experienced (Park & Folkman, 1997). Traumatic events may shatter a person's worldview and self identity (Fife, 1994; Janoff-Bulman & Berg, 1998). The balance is abruptly altered, which creates disharmony in one's existence. The process of cognitive reappraisal of the traumatic event, searching for meaning, and the integration of the experience into one's life schema help people to adapt to the losses brought about by the event (Lazarus & Folkman, 1984.; Taylor, 1983). The reconstruction of meaning after loss involves the process of "sense making," "benefit finding," and "identity reconstruction" (Davies, Nolen-Hoeksema, & Larson, 1998; Neimeyer, 2000; Neimeyer, Prigerson, & Davies, 2002). We engage clients in a process of re-storying their lives in developing more coherent narratives of their experiences. We help them to discover their gains in suffering. We find that the concepts of impermanence and unpredictability of life from Buddhism and Daoism are very useful in helping clients to re-construct their loss experience and make sense of their misery. The critical review in the narrative process will inevitably lead to the reappraisal of the meaning of the self, the family and, ultimately, life. The fundamental values and philosophies of the client will be critically revisited, and reconstructed if necessary. The deliberation is not limited to the client's intrinsic world. It also emphasizes the relationship between the client and the environment-the social and natural world. This helps the client to regain the necessary fluidity and balance of existence.

In our infertility counseling project at the assisted reproduction clinic of our teaching hospital, we see many couples under immense stress. At the surface level, the stress is induced by the medical procedure, which is torturous with a success rate of only about one in four. At the deeper level, it is related to their fixated value on the meaning of the self, family, and life. We facilitate a critical revisiting and reconstruction of these values. By letting go of control, such as thinking "we must have children in our family or life" and "we must succeed in assisted reproduction", they regain control of themselves and their lives. This is the true cure of the stress because it deals with the underlying issue. The couples find new meaning in their families and their lives, and can get along whatever the outcome of the assisted reproduction process. This approach is fundamentally different from many infertility counseling practices in the West that regard stress reduction as the means to an end - i.e. enhancing compliance and to continue with assisted reproduction procedures. We are afraid that such an instrumental stress reduction approach is itself stress inducing.

Appreciation: This aims at fostering a renewed appreciation of life. Appreciation is grounded in full acceptance, but is more than that. It is not simply an absence of negatives, but is about the presence of positives. The motto of the Society for the Promotion of Hospice Care in Hong Kong is *"when days cannot be added to life, add life to days."* This promotes a proactive attitude in fully and truly living every day.

Most psychosocial intervention models deliver the treatment sequentially, most notably increasing the depth of intervention as the treatment makes progress. A core characteristic of our Body-Mind-Spirit approach is that we deliver our intervention in a circular manner. Spiritual issues are included in our first session with clients. This approach is necessary and coherent with our belief in the interconnectedness of the body, mind, and spirit. Our clinical experience tells us that the approach works well and speeds up the healing process. Most of our therapeutic groups take only about four to five sessions to complete. Hence, we need to emphasize that although the interventions in the body, mind, and spiritual domains are presented in a sequential manner in this paper, in the actual clinical process they are delivered in a spiral manner, right from the first encounter with the clients.

CONCLUSION

This paper advocates a positive, transformation-oriented perspective in working with clients who are experiencing major difficulties in life. While the more traditional, psychopathology-oriented approach may be content with symptom reduction and adaptive functioning, we aim at going beyond survivorship. Inspired by holistic model of Chinese Medicine, we develop the Eastern body-mind-spirit approach with the primary therapy goal of facilitating harmonious dynamic equilibrium within oneself, as well as between oneself and the natural and social environment. To achieve this, multimodal interventions are employed, including vitalizing body work, such as simplified Tai Chi and Qigong exercises, acupressure, body scan, breathing meditation, and mindful tea drinking and eating, as well as vibrant mind and spirit process, such as the acknowledgement and acceptance of impermanence and unpredictability, regaining self-control by letting go of control, the appreciation and affirmation of life, and fostering loving-kindness and forgiveness. The creative multimodal interventions can activate the interconnected body-mind-spirit system to rebalance itself and arrive at a new harmonious dynamic equilibrium.

After more than 10 years of trials on various clienteles and repeated efficacy evaluations, we feel confident in claiming that our approach works and has some merit. Being strength-focused, we can activate and connect with clients at an amazingly quick pace. With a multimodal intervention, we can engage a wider range of clients, including those who are uncomfortable with articulating their thinking and emotions verbally.

Being growth and transformation oriented, we witness wonders and changes in many of our clients. Some of them become devoted to helping others and building a better world for all. In face of suffering, we have many choices—we can fight, flee, or seek haven in some form of psychological defense. Following traditional Chinese wisdom, we advocate an alternative that is neither fight nor flight. Suffering is suffering, but no more than that. We can accept it, live with it, be at peace with it, and achieve a new harmonious equilibrium. Thereby we gain deeper insight into the meaning of life through suffering. That is transformation.

NOTES

1. Since the Second World War, Western medicine has evolved from a conventional biological model toward a more holistic approach in care, as witnessed by the notable developments in social psychiatry, family medicine, mind-body medicine, and integrative medicine.

2. The Theory of the Five Elements is an ancient Chinese systems framework for the understanding of balance, harmony, and change. First, it proposes that all things in the world can be classified by the Five Elements. Second, there is a universal pattern of change and dynamic relationship among the broad categories. Third, by applying the knowledge of the universal model, one can understand the change pattern among the items being investigated, for example, the inter-relationships among various organs, emotions, and thoughts of a person. The Five Elements denote wood, fire, earth, metal, and water, which represent five broad categories. There are two normal forces—the facilitating force and the repressing force—working on each other among the elements. Wood facilitates fire, fire facilitates earth, earth facilitates metal, metal facilitates water, and water facilitates wood. Meanwhile, wood represses earth, fire represses metal, earth represses water, metal represses wood, and water represses fire. The two forces working together maintain the dynamic equilibrium among the five elements, without any one becoming "hypo" or "hyper". Harmonious, fluid balance is regarded as the healthy state.

According to this classification scheme, the five organs are liver, heart, spleen, lung, and kidney; and the five emotions are anger, joy, worry, sorrow, and fear. Extreme anger will harm the liver. Hypermania can hurt the heart. Having too much worry will affect the digestive system (spleen). Sorrow can affect health of the lungs. Being fearful can affect the functions of the kidney and reproductive systems.

REFERENCES

Abramson, R. J. (2003). The unity of mind, body, and spirit: A five element view of cancer. *Advances in Mind-Body Medicine, 19*(2), 20–21.

Baer, R. A. (2003). Mindfulness training as a clinical intervention: A conceptual and empirical review. *Clinical Psychology: Science and Practice, 10*(2), 125–143.

Beinfield, H., & Korngold. (2003). Chinese medicine and cancer care. *Alternative Therapies in Health and Medicine, Sep/Oct, 9*(5), p. 38–52.

Bensoussan, A., & Talley, N. J. (1998). Treatment of Irritable Bowel Syndrome With Chinese Herbal Medicine: A Randomized Controlled Trial. *JAMA, 280* (1585), 1–11.

Bonanno, G. A. (2004). Loss, trauma, and human resilience: Have we underestimated the human capacity to thrive after extremely aversive events? *American Psychologist, 59*(1), 20–28.

Cai, J. (1995). *Advanced Textbook on Traditional Chinese Medicine and Pharmacology Vol. 1.* Beijing: New World Press.

Chan, C. L. W. (2001). *An Eastern Body-Mind-Spirit Approach - A training manual with one-second techniques.* Hong Kong: Department of Social Work & Social Administration, The University of Hong Kong.

Chan, C. L. W., Ho, P. S. Y., & Chow, E. (2001). A body-mind-spirit model in health: an eastern approach. *Social Work in Health Care, 34*(3/4), 261–282.

Davies, C. G., Nolen-Hoeksema, S., & Larson, J. (1998). Making sense of loss and benefiting from the experience: Two construals of meaning. *Journal of Personality and Social Psychology, 75*(2), 561–574.

Engel, G. L. (1977). The need for a new medical model: a challenge for biomedicine. *Science, 196*(4286), 129–136.

Fife, B. L. (1994). The conceptualization of meaning in illness. *Social Science & Medicine, 38*(2), 309–316.

Friedman, H. S. (2002). *Health Psychology* (2nd ed.). New Jersey: Prentice Hall.

Green, J., & Shellenberger, R. (1991). *The dynamics of health and wellness: A biopsychosocial approach.* Fort Worth: Harcourt Brace College Publishers.

Ho, S. M. Y., Chan, C. L. W., & Ho, R. T. H. (2004). Posttraumatic growth in Chinese cancer survivors. *Psycho-oncology, 13*(6), 377–389.

Hung, D. G. (1993). *Essence of Qigong.* Hong Kong: Tiendi Publishing House.

Huppert, F. A., & Whittington, J. (2003). Evidence for the independence of positive and negative well-being: Implications for quality of life assessment. *British Journal of Health Psychology, 8*, 107–122.

Janoff-Bulman, R., & Berg, M. (1998). Disillusionment and the creation of values. In H. Harvey (Ed.), *Perspectives on loss.* New York: Brunner/Mazel.

Lao-zi. (6th century B.C.). *Tao Te Ching. Annotated by W. H. Chan (1st ed.).* Hong Kong: Commercial Press (in Chinese).

Lazarus, R. S., & Folkman, S. (1984). *Stress, appraisal, and coping.* New York: Springer Publishing Co.

Li, K. K., & Yang, B. F. (1999). *Lecture Notes of the Essence of Golden Cabinet.* Shanghai: Shanghai Science & Technology Publishing House (in Chinese).

Neimeyer, R. A. (2000). Searching for the meaning of meaning: Grief therapy and the process of reconstruction. *Death Studies, 24*(Issue 6), 541–559.

Neimeyer, R. A., Prigerson, H. G., & Davies, B. (2002). Mourning and meaning. *American Behavioral Scientist, 46*, 235–251.

Ng, S. M. (2003). *Chinese Medicine Yangsheng and Body/Mind/Spirit Wellness.* Hong Kong: Veritas Book House (in Chinese).

Ogden, J. (2000). *Health Psychology: A textbook* (2nd ed.). Philadelphia: Open University Press.

Pachuta, D. M. (1989). Chinese medicine: The law of five elements. In A. A. Sheikh & K. S. Sheikh (Eds.), *Eastern and Western approaches to healing: Ancient wisdom and modern knowledge* (pp. 64–90). New York: John Wiley & Sons.

Park, C. L. (1998). Stress-related growth and thriving through coping: The roles of personality and cognitive processes. *Journal of Social Issues, 54*(2), 211–267

Park, C. L., & Folkman, S. (1997). Meaning in the Context of Stress and Coping. *Review of General Psychology, 1*(2), 115–144.

Seligman, M. E., & Csikszentmihalyi, M. (2000). Positive Psychology: An Introduction. *American Psychologist, 55*(1), 5–14.

Taylor, S. (1983). Adjustment to threatening events: a cognitive theory of adaptation. *American Psychologist, 38*, 1161–1173.

Tedeschi, R. G., & Calhoun, L. G. (1996). The Posttraumatic Growth Inventory: Measuring the positive legacy of trauma. *Journal of Trauma Stress, 9*, 455–471.

Wang, H. T., Chiu, M. S., & Hong, P. (2000). *Selected Readings from the Inner Canon of Chinese Medicine.* Shanghai: Shanghai Science & Technology Publishing House (in Chinese).

WHO. (2002). *WHO Traditional Medicine Stratgy.* Geneva: World Health Organization.

Wong, B., & McKeen, J. (1998). *The New Manual for Life.* Vancouver: PD Publishing.

Yin, H. H., Zhang, B. L., Zhang, C. Y., Zhang, S. C., & Meng, S. M. (1994). *Foundations of Chinese medicine.* Shanghai: Shanghai Scientific (in Chinese).

A Critical Approach to Pedagogy in Mental Health

Marty Dewees, PhD, LICSW
Lisa K. Lax, MSW, LICSW

"I'm not mental. You can see that. I don't understand why my son left. I want my boy back. I'm not incompetent. Life can make you incompetent. If there's no roof over your heard, it can make you depressed."

Gondolf, 1998, p. 50

"'She's really faking it,' is the psychiatrist's appraisal of Judy's semiconscious behavior through the interview. The 25-year-old black woman is brought into the emergency room slouched in a wheel chair, shabbily dressed, and without shoes, and apparently in a deep sleep. It is the patient's third overdose using alcohol and Valium."

Gondolf, 1998, p. 55

The messages in the forsaken voices remind us that the mental health system in the United States is characterized by competing and untidy demands. In the emergency room, the urban clinic, and the rural community mental health center, people come for help who are poor, disorganized, beaten, or apparently swallowed up by adversity. Their providers are likewise compassionate, overworked, and suspicious, burned out, helpful, and sometimes at a loss to help in a system increasingly influenced by medical and legal constructs. How can social workers make sense of these scenarios? How can they make a difference?

Western culture has constructed "mental health" as an individualized medical issue that is constitutionally situated in one's "proprietary space," or in the usual metaphor, "head." Further, our system of care is based on the conviction that indicators of mental health belong to a unitary, internally focused framework, conceived by medicine and codified in the psychiatric nomenclature of the *Diagnostic and Statistical Manual of Mental Disorders, Text Revision (DSM-IV-TR)* (American Psychiatric Association, 2000). This article explores the connections between social work and mental health, the nature of social work practice in the contemporary mental health service system, and the tasks of social work educators in the preparation of practitioners. Next, it proposes a critical approach to teaching mental health that emphasizes social work's distinctiveness and its traditional focus on relationship and person-in-environment as it plays out in the postmodern world. Finally, the authors include sample student assignments and exercises that demonstrate this pedagogical approach.

THE INTERFACE OF SOCIAL WORK AND MENTAL HEALTH

Social workers constitute the largest group of mental health professionals and mental health is the largest field of practice in the profession (Bentley & Taylor, 2002). This should render social work's voice in mental health as unique, with a clear sense of identity and an abiding commitment to its legacy of social justice, human rights, and advocacy. Yet, social workers in many corners of mental health practice have displaced the profession's mission of social justice (Hoff, Huff, & Ord, 1996; Specht & Courtney, 1994) in exchange for the language, trappings, and goals that reflect our particular culture's admiration of medicine. This is partly because medicine in Western cultures carries more prestige than many professions (Dewees, 2002) and social workers have gained status by attaching themselves to it, as well as adopting parallel tracts for training, licensure, and reimbursement. It is also likely that the field's traditional occupation by women has contributed to its modest stature among the professions and that its "combination of pragmatism and caring" (Weick, 1999, p. 327) translates into "less" somehow than the more scientific, objective, and distant profiles that medicine and psychiatry have traditionally adopted. Social work's location in the mental health system, then, puts it in a curious bind. The profession takes a central place within a constellation that focuses on the individual and the isolated, inner life of the mind while at the same time its very core is tied to relationship and context. The following explores this phenomenon in the realm of social work practice in mental health.

THE DISCONNECT BETWEEN INDIVIDUALISM AND SOCIAL WORK PRACTICE

In the dominant contemporary practice context of mental health services, many social work practitioners play an increasingly medicalized role as they are called upon to formulate diagnoses based on the *DSM-IV-TR*, a psychiatric rather than social work framework. For example, in school settings, social workers are often required to diagnose 5-year-olds in order to fund social services to them (see Kutchins & Kirk, 1988). In such procedures, the emphasis is firmly planted in individual attributes which are interpreted as pathological, whether they arise from psychobiology, intrapsychic stressors, troubled relationships, or problematic structural dynamics, such as poverty.

But what of social work's traditional person-in-environment focus? How does the social work purpose play out in the "real" world? As social workers explore clients' lived experiences and trace their impact, they may begin to question the focus of their professional attention. The authors will consider a selected cross section of contexts that frequently frame the experiences of those who see or are compelled to receive help in contemporary practice in the global world of the 21st century. These areas include (1) domestic and sexual violence, (2) oppression, and (3) global interdependence. Three among many, all interface with the mental health system in ways that emerge as challenging for social work practice.

Domestic and Sexual Violence

A compelling and ever-expanding area of practice, the work against domestic and sexual violence has frequently collided with the mental health system (Gondolf, 1998). There are many reasons for this, but one of the most enduring appears to be the deep-seated differences in worldviews between the indigenous, grass-roots movement emerging from the feminist community to oppose violence against women and the professional, medicalized lens of individualism born of psychiatry (Warshaw, 2003).

The intersection with mental health. The primary impasse occurs when the systems addressing violence and mental health intersect. Antiviolence advocates are likely to hold the view that violence is a *social*, interactive issue, born of and sustained in societal assumptions regarding gender and/ or power relations. Accordingly, survivors may present with many behaviors that are seen as originating in or exacerbated by the violence they have experienced. Behavioral manifestations of fear, loss, disillusionment, and mistrust may be interpreted as part of the *social* sequelae of intimate partner violence. These behaviors may include self-destructive gestures, withdrawal, unwillingness to engage, outbursts of rage, accusations of malice, or obliteration of consciousness through substance use.

These same issues of conduct may be interpreted by mental health professionals as clear and pathological symptoms of paranoia, borderline personality disorder, mania, or depression. Coping measures and survival strategies may be seen as further evidence of disorder (Warshaw, Moroney, & Barnes, 2003). When these are framed as *DSM* syndromes with predictable and categorical symptoms, they act as assignations of individual mental, character, and personality flaws. The short-term goal then is symptom control or relief while the longer range hope is for adjustment of the dynamic in the interactive, interpersonal couple system that supports the violence. The individual survivor and aggressor are the key change agents and the broader social system continues unabated and unchallenged.

The challenge for social work. This particular intersection is sometimes sticky for social workers in mental health. Clinicians trained in traditional mental health models along with a person-in-environment focus may find themselves pulled between views of how the world goes. The components of social justice and human rights, strong bedrock principles for social workers, confound the conundrum. "Person-in-environment" does not imply an impartial playing field in which all members must simply adapt to achieve harmony. Inevitably, person-in-environment, in a postmodern and global world, mandates the consideration of power and its dynamics. A simple analysis of our patriarchal society suggests that the dynamic between, for example, a woman and her male partner often does not fit into the egalitarian "you-get-what-you-give" philosophy implied in the tenets of many family systems models. A commitment to human rights and social justice then, will complicate the medicalization of violence and lead to its formulation as a complex *social* phenomenon rather than a matter of individual weakness, interpersonal incompatibility, bad temper, or pathology.

Social workers in practice hear the sometimes paralyzing stories and see the devastating legacy of violence on survivor's lives and those of their children. Because they are trained to evaluate and experience the context, they are frequently challenged to sort out the mental health aspects from those of violence. It can't be done. Violence is an egregious threat to mental health and it is both an intensely personal and a politically systematized issue. Social workers in antiviolence work who also value and are committed particularly to the rights of women all over the world can find little, if any, cold solace in an intricately tuned diagnosis of psychopathology.

Oppression

In spite of the wealth and privilege of contemporary western cultures, social workers are no strangers to oppression. Violations of basic human rights and other forms of injustice create tensions every day in their professional and personal lives. Listening to the stories of people of color, people with disabilities, and people with alternative sexual orientations offers perspectives that differ from the dominant white, ablest, heterosexual mode. Social workers are also trained to notice correlations in the rates of poverty and ethnic or class "difference." They bear witness to acts of cruelty and injustice that "other" people encounter. Hopefully, they note the power of the malevolence of these experiences as well as the harmful impact of turning some people inward thus killing the spirit to become the promise of their early dreams.

The medicalization of racism. Social workers try to make sense of this. They may refer to "autoppressors" (Lieberman, p. 85) or "internalized oppression" (Pheterson, p. 35) when the person referred for help seems to accept and become the prejudiced picture painted by oppressors. They may label it "poor self esteem" or "weak ego" as they approach psychiatric territory in their language. Jackson (2002) notes in a powerful narrative of African-American experience in the white mental health system that Benjamin Rush, the erstwhile "father of American psychiatry" who lived in the late 18th century, coined a condition called "Negritude" which was used to explain the insanity that some Africans developed soon after entering slavery. Thought to be a form of leprosy, as Jackson tells it, Negritude had only one, highly improbable cure—to become white (Jackson, p. 14).

The US has a long and well-established history of systematic oppression. Its very borders were appropriated through acts that were both aggressive against and exploitive of Native Americans and Alaska natives. In the course of the following years, through a Civil War and two world wars, through exploitation, attempts to secure cheap labor, and through a host of unjust practices, many ethnic minorities have been placed into a world of persistent poverty and discrimination. The repercussions of such practices have made their way into the mental health system. Oppressed people apparently have psychiatric attributes that are divergent from those of the dominant culture. Today African men, particularly, may be seen as "aggressive" or "menacing" (for example see "You may keep the yacht" in Spitzer, Gibbon, Skodol, & First, 1994, p. 67).

As social workers explore the implications of mental health treatment for African Americans and other ethnicities of color, they find, at the very least, that the system has routinely and substantially mismanaged psychiatric treatment through misdiagnosis, more severe diagnoses than symptoms warranted, and less treatment than whites received (Davis, 2001; Sands, 2001).

Inappropriate solutions. All of the above situational factors reflect, just as those inherent in domestic and sexual violence, a worldview of the individual as a unitary mix of independent perception, cognition, personality, and disposition, shaped by genetic and physical environmental factors but bereft of the *social*. Social work practitioners recognize, however, the reciprocal nature of oppression. For every "internalized oppression" there is an "internalized domination" (Pheterson, 1999, p. 35) producing arrogance, feelings of superiority, normalcy, and self righteousness (among other things) in members of the dominant group. What of these? What is the profession's path in recognizing the person-in-environment when the environment is so shaped by these perceptions? How do these impact the mental health status of those who experience oppression?

The absurdity of Rush's solution for the "condition" he called "Negritude" clearly demonstrates the twisted inapplicability, now generally construed in more sophisticated terms, of an individual focus for so many of the populations social workers serve in the practice context. The voice of social work has to reflect a simple logic here: if the "affliction" is born of oppression, then oppression has to be addressed. To be sure, the solution is not simple, but to analyze, diagnose, and "treat" the survival of oppression as an individual deficit defies commonsense as well as the human rights commitments of the profession.

Global Interdependence

Western nations, particularly the US, have tended to be myopic about the connectedness of the world (Healy, 2001). In whatever ways most people long for the haven of their homes, neighborhoods, states, or nations, social workers need to recognize the responsibilities and the opportunities that are inherent in the contemporary global world. Healy suggests at least fours ways in which current, everyday social work is impacted by this interdependence. These have to do with: (1) migration patterns, (2) world widespread social conditions, (3) the systems effects of one country's actions on others, and (4) the advent of technology. The authors will look very briefly at each of these interrelated phenomena to examine the connections between them and social work practice in mental health.

Migration patterns. The international social, political, and economic events of war, globalized economics, and the struggle for power have created migration patterns all over the world. These have resulted in the devastating dislocation dynamics of refugee status for millions and have created complex transborder issues with regard to protection and human rights. Western social workers cannot hide behind national boundaries here. Social workers in most major cities in the US and in many rural areas as well are likely to confront these issues in everyday practice, as, for example, a family of non-English-speaking, possession-less, refugees is resettled into a heartland community. Social workers must carefully consider differing cultural contexts and meanings in their practice as they recognize and work with people from one culture struggling to find a place in another so vastly different. In such situations it will not be helpful to prioritize DSM depictions of individual "depression," (when a service user's family has been annihilated, lost, or starved to death) or "adjustment disorders" (in adolescents attempting to come to terms with, say, youth culture in the middle of Ohio). Social isolation, loss of community, and disruption of "important life projects" are identified as major stressors in the experience of exile (Miller et al., 2002) and requires a "new paradigm in mental health care"—and a holistic, community-focused understanding of the "broader social policy contexts in which refugees are placed" (Watters, 2001, p. 1709).

Worldwide social conditions. The shared agenda of widespread social conditions around the world such as homelessness, poverty, violence, street children, increasing longevity, to name only a few, knows no borders. Western social workers have typically seen their models as exports to be adopted by other nations. This is no longer an adequate response. Western social work's preoccupation with "remedial" models (Midgley, 1999), which by definition are individualistic and meant to cure, is not a strategy that nations of the Global South can afford, nor is it appropriate. As structural issues borne by individuals, these conditions can be addressed only indirectly and piecemeal in current, often medicalized, efforts to eradicate symptoms or comfort the miserable. Although there will always be a place for face-to-face response to individual pain, one of social work's major roles should be to facilitate planned social change and economic development that will provide the conditions in which individual and collective mental health can flourish. The person-in-environment lens must attend to a sophisticated understanding of "environment" within a global focus.

Systemic effects. As citizens, social workers now know, rather more acutely than they would prefer, how the actions of one country can alter the course of another's. The events of September 11, 2001 will remain sharply etched in the minds of most US citizens for a long time. The thoughtful among us will ponder the provocations for such an attack and the hatred that inspired it. In turn, social workers can think through how this phenomenon has reshaped their political grounding, their current conceptions of civil rights, and their analysis of the components of freedom. These are not individual issues. Even while social workers offer individual counseling for adjustment and support to victims and families for grief issues, their larger view is on the status of just global relationships, and the meanings of poverty, disenfranchisement, and alienation in places across the world as they affect the mental health of all citizens.

The advent of technology. Finally, the enormous advent and growth of technology in the last 20 years has left the world a different place. Communications as an industry has changed the course of nearly all cultures, from the most teeming urban centers to tiny villages in countries that westerners have never heard of. The opportunity to share perspectives and approaches is so pervasive in contemporary society that social workers clearly cannot afford to rest smugly with their individualized treatment approaches. Only western social workers tend to use such remedial models and individual services, while others look to community frameworks for social development (Rowe, Hanley, Moreno, & Mould, 2000). Social workers need to reach out, for example, to cultures in which there is no such recognized beast as a personality disorder and they need to explore, among other phenomena, lifelong oppression as a genesis of paranoia. They need to define mental health in terms of human community and focus on the threats to its potential. In the global world, these appear to reside in the fortresses of poverty, oppression, disease, hopelessness, and futureless children.

Implications for Social Work Education

What is the role, then, of the social work educator in this context? The general task of professional education is the preparation of practitioners. All professions have grounding in theory and perspective and all also change, as they are reflections of the sociocultural context. Social work is no exception. It would seem, then, that social work educators need to train their students to assume positions in the current culture of the profession. In addition, they need to model and sustain a vision for what the profession could become in the future. This requires that educators teach both content and critique as they consider what they want to contribute to students entering the field.

Multilingual Content

The concept of multilingualism is helpful in integrating the many discourses that students encounter. They will need to think in and speak several languages. They will have already learned the traditional social work language in their early course work and will probably be fluent in "person-in-environment speak." They will likely have background in systems and ecosystems theory or ecological approaches to viewing practice context. There are many well-known approaches to these, such as the Generalist Intervention Model (GIM) (Kirst-Ashman & Hull, 2002), the ecosystems/problem-solving focus (Compton & Galaway, 1999), and the direct practice/ecological approach (Hepworth, Rooney, & Larsen (2001), to name only a few.

It is likely that many of the perspectives in this language will include some quasi–mental-health terminology like "treatment," "resistance," or "therapist" that has been generated from the profession's flirtation with psychiatric models. Many of these have become time-honored and are now seen as part of social work. A case can be made that they are indeed a part of social work, since the profession's tenets and the language that reflects them evolve as do all living things. Therefore, the question of what is or is not "truly" social work, reflected in which language, will often be moot.

Nevertheless, it is important to examine the language social workers use and how it shapes the way they think. If there is inquiry for instance, regarding whether coursework in graduate programs is promoting a critical approach to social work practice in mental health (see, for example, Lacasse & Gomory, 2003), one might chose to look beyond courses entitled "psychopathology." The term itself intimates the adoption of a discourse that is a relatively poor fit, if not downright inimical, to many of social work's current critical, theoretical perspectives in which more liberating positions are focal points.

Given, then, that there are varied idioms within social work, educators will want to assist students in their capacity to understand, engage in dialogue and critique the ones most relevant to them. To that end, three important content representations of the discourse of mental health are explored.

The DSM. The DSM, as a single icon, is the most representative and arguably most controversial component of the practice discourse in the US mental health system. The literature has for many years reflected lively debate on its merits as science, its relevance to social work practice, and its usefulness in social work education (see Kirk & Kutchins, 1992; Kirk & Kutchins, 1994; Kutchins & Kirk. 1995; Kirk & Kutchins, 1997; Williams & Spitzer, 1995). However one views these questions, it remains a fact that the DSM continues to be the major reference for the classification of mental illnesses and the legitimation of mental health services. Both its use and diagnostic dominion in managed and behavioral health care schemes, which currently pervade the mental health landscape, have only expanded over the most recent years.

In this arena, social work educators cannot afford to dismiss the relevance of the *DSM* to their students. They needn't embrace its science, philosophy, or implications, but they need to teach about them. Students need to be prepared for the world they will enter, and, most important, they need the tools to engage in the struggle for changing it. One cannot critique what one doesn't know.

Theory. There are, of course, a host of theories generating from all corners of the helping professions. No social worker or educator will know them all, but it is important for students to gain some facility with those that are both most frequently used (e.g., cognitive behavioral, psychodynamic) and which also offer the most hopefulness for effective, values-consistent practice. While the intent here is not to be prescriptive, in the authors' view(s) that list would include:

1. narrative theory, in which the central focus is on the participant's story;
2. feminist theories, in which there is analysis of power according to gender;
3. empowerment theory, in which the focus is on unleashing potential; and
4. relational-cultural theory, in which connections and relationships are highlighted, rather than separation and independence.

The importance of theory here lies in its *application* to both the individually focused conceptualizations used in the mental health system and the more contextually and experientially oriented perspectives generated in social work and other related fields. Understanding the theoretical influences on practice can be invaluable in evaluating and critiquing its repercussions on the lives of the people social workers serve. For example, a Freudian theoretical analysis that conceptualizes a battered woman as, for example, struggling with unconscious, unresolved intrapsychic conflict, is likely to lead to a very different approach to the work than a more empowerment-oriented or relational stance would suggest.

Standpoint. "Standpoint" as a theoretical perspective literally refers to the idea that our reality depends on "where we stand" (Lieberman, 1998). As such the positions practitioners take in practice (as in life) are grounded in the perceptions that emerge from their places in society. These "places" take form within a context of race, gender, class, history, and status. Professional views of any practice context, theory, or participant are shaped by all of the experiences and attributes brought to the work. Students may need explicit assistance with this idea to recognize, for example, that because of their positions in society, they are likely in some circumstances to trust "authority" or "professionalism" without questioning their repercussions for others or even themselves. In other scenarios workers might dismiss new or unorthodox approaches automatically because they don't fit the traditional positions that emerge from their standpoints. Since what human beings consider "real" is based on their particular place of grounding, social workers must be acutely attuned to their own standpoints, as well as those of others.

The importance of understanding standpoint rests in recognition of the implications it has for assessment and evaluation. For example, if US practitioners value assertiveness, independence, and achievement, they may view a Hopi child's culturally sanctioned reluctance to compete against his peers or question his elders as a sign of slowness, poor self esteem, withdrawal, developmental delay, or even depression. It is the *function* of standpoint here, as distinguished from the *content*, with which students need explicit experience.

Dialogic Critique

There are many ways in which social work professionals critique their work. In a world of individualized practice in a managed care environment, they are likely to look to quantitative, empirical measures evidencing successful change. They might also consider outcomes reflecting client-generated values like completing school or staying out of trouble with the law, and they might even inquire about client satisfaction. But social workers in a system in which there is constant tension between the medical and the social will also want to engage in a sustained, dialogic process with colleagues and others to consider some key questions that go beyond immediate client outcomes. Two of these follow.

Who benefits from this approach to the work? This critical inquiry goes beyond individual achievement of change. Social workers need to question who benefits from the centrality of the *DSM* and who benefits from the diagnostic procedure. The repercussions of diagnosis, including a consideration of stigma and how this influences the lives of the people with whom they work are important points of critical examination. How does diagnosis assist *social workers* in working with the relational issues inherent in domestic and sexual violence, oppression, and global interdependence? How should socials workers respond to this kind of classification in those contexts?

Social workers committed to critical reflection in their practice must also be aware of and question the influence of theoretical perspectives. Is repression of unconscious inner conflict, for example, a useful lens through which to view people experiencing violence at the hands of intimate partners or dominant cultures? How can practitioners address the dimensions of relatedness that their clients experience in the phenomena of violence and oppression?

Social workers should also assess their own standpoints in relation to those of their clients and examine the implication of these upon their work. Do they enhance or impede clients' progress? For example, does the standpoint of a white, middle-class worker who tends to avoid conflict affect the way he or she works with an angry, young Hispanic who is being discriminated against in the workplace? How might such a worker evaluate her "disruptive" behavior? What kind of diagnosis might be made? Whose standpoint might it reflect?

How do practice approaches fit with professional values? Social work has always placed the highest priority on its values. On the most basic level these have to do with human rights and a respect for the dignity of all people, not just members of the articulate worried well, and not just the introspective and verbal, but all people. In the mental health system sometimes clients are dirty, angry, belligerent, smell bad, and seem to live in world others don't recognize as real. Sometimes they are grandiose, sometimes they hurt others, and they don't always appreciate the opportunity to work with professionals. How do practitioners' approaches to them and their work with them highlight the dignity to which social workers are committed? How are human rights supported by the DSM? Is it a culture-free tool? Is it blind to privilege? How do theories fit with the values of worth and self direction? Where do the positions of workers, born from their standpoints, conflict with the profession's values?

The purpose of teaching and advocating for this kind of critique with students is not to negate the usefulness of a medicalized view of mental health that may be appropriate for a psychiatric approach to individual symptoms. It is rather to promote a *social work* response that sustains the profession's grounding. These and other like questions help students to develop a truly critical view of their practice in mental health which they can take with them from graduate school and apply throughout their careers. They no doubt develop other mechanisms for this kind of critique, as well, and certainly are constantly exposed to additional and dynamic content. In the following section, the authors will demonstrate some of the methods they use with students to consider these themes.

PEDAGOGICAL EXAMPLES

In order to bring these ideas to life, the authors have developed a series of exercises for student use in the classroom. The following represents a sampling of these. Each group addresses one of the dimensions of the multilingual content (DSM, theory, and standpoint) described above, as it is integrated with the two processes of dialogic critique just considered.

Diagnosis in Context (DSM)

Social work students enrolled in mental health courses are invariably faced with written case studies in which a mythical or actual client's presenting issues and symptoms are described. These descriptions allow students to practice their skills in categorization and assessment. Typically, these studies do not include much in the way of contextual information, preserving, as they do, an individual, internal lens. Students tend to focus on "getting the diagnosis right" by matching details in a study with symptom descriptions outlined in the DSM. The challenge for social work educators is to facilitate learning about the accurate use of diagnostic nosology while helping students keep a firm grounding in social work's emphasis on social and environmental context. An additional challenge is to encourage students to think about diagnosis as a method best put "in brackets," so that it does not privilege their professional knowledge or shape the ways in which they listen to the stories of their clients (Hartman, 1994).

One exercise designed to facilitate this synthesis involves separating symptoms from contextual information. In class, group A is given a case description with an emphasis on symptoms and presenting problems. Group B is given the same description but with an added paragraph about the person's interpersonal and social circumstances. Each group deliberates on its respective client description separately and then the two groups come back together to share their differing assessments, diagnoses, and intervention approaches.

Example 1: Mrs. H, a woman in her 50s, presents at a rural mental health clinic with persistent depressed mood, irritability, distrust, extreme isolation, and reports a history of multiple psychiatric hospitalizations.

Contextual detail informs students of her long history of sexual and physical abuse in her marriage and her decision to divorce her husband after her most recent involuntary hospitalization which was based on false information given by her husband to the designated screeners in her community. Her husband continues to live in the small community and has described Mrs. H to others as "crazy."

Example 2: A mail room employee in a business organization is referred to an Employee Assistance Program counselor for problems on the job with anger and difficulty getting along with coworkers. In the interview, he appears withdrawn and anxious. He complains of a variety of physical ailments, including stomach problems and headaches. He distrusts his supervisor and is angry about the referral.

Contextual detail informs students that this African American man is the only person of color employed by a small local company in a rural state. He has been experiencing harassment from his coworkers for months and feels trapped to stay because there is no other employment available to him in the community. He has not reported the harassment to anyone in the company because he watched a lesbian coworker be harassed and fired after she complained.

In both examples, contextual information shapes the assessment process and alters perceptions about diagnosis. Further, students are given the opportunity to evaluate whether psychiatric diagnosis is relevant at all in these case studies and to consider interventions that do not fit under the traditional mental health rubric of "treatment" but are more consistent with the profession's stance on social justice and human rights. Case studies such as these can lead to discussion regarding who benefits from transforming such experiences of personal violation into individual pathologies.

Critical Application of Theory

In agency-based field placements, social work students engaged in mental health practice are exposed to theory through treatment approaches used by their host agencies. Most often these are the approaches favored by managed care organizations or government funding sources, which may or may not be grounded in empirically based outcome studies. Practice approaches informed by particular theories might have evolved in an agency as "best practice" over time and are often presented and taught uncritically to students. In the authors' experience, it is common for students to be unaware of which theoretical model informs an approach being used in their practice. A written assignment designed to help students identify, then analyze, a particular approach encourages critical thinking and a "disciplined eclecticism" (see Roche, 2004) approach to the use of theory in social work practice.

In one assignment, students are asked to write a paper in which they first describe a case situation in their practice, their assessment, and choice of diagnosis. They are then asked to identify, describe, and critically analyze the theoretical model and practice approach utilized, drawing from their assessment of the strengths, shortcomings, and the implications of the theoretical stance for the client. Finally, they are asked to identify an alternative model which would address concerns identified in the critique and to describe how this alternative model would alter their practice and results. The intent is for students to "play with" theory, develop an understanding of how theory influences practice, and to gain experience and comfort with the critical examination of theory in their own work as helpers.

Situating One's Position in Standpoint

In social work certain stances, or positions, may be comfortable and therefore often go unquestioned. For example, assumed positions such as "involuntary treatment should be abolished" or "labeling people dehumanizes" are consistent with the sentiments of many social workers and thus they are easily adopted by students in social work programs. Opposing positions on the same issues, while less comfortable, are also valuable to consider because they require a greater commitment to critical thinking. Further, positions that concern human behavior and attributes and are deeply rooted in dominant cultural views can be even more challenging to deconstruct for many of the (usually) middle-class social work students in the US. Three exercises that explore these issues are described below.

To facilitate recognition and awareness of the repercussions of their own standpoints which include cultural, class, and ethnic biases, students are first asked to assume the standpoint of an "other" person from a different culture, class, or race from which to view a mental health issue. For example, students are asked to research and to take a position on mandated substance abuse treatment requiring weekly individual therapy and sporadic urine screens from the perspective or standpoint of someone from a Native American culture which embraces communal and spiritual healing practices. Additionally, the student is asked to view the same issue from the standpoint of a culturally main stream corrections officer with a responsibility to monitor court mandated treatment. Here students discuss how these standpoints are likely to influence the positions taken in the work and what implications they might have for clients.

Reflecting the issue from a slightly different perspective, students are then assigned a position on a mental health issue, for example, the use of disability benefits. One position on such benefits reflects the conviction that it is imperative for all immigrants and refugees to work to support themselves. Students then consider this position and its implications from two different perspectives: first, from the standpoint of a Vietnamese refugee with a mental illness and a strong work ethic; and second, from the standpoint of a US-born, economically privileged, community mental health center case manager with a strong caring ethic. Here again, students can explore the effects of standpoint on both clients and providers.

A third exercise uses a case example in which an agency decides to locate a residential treatment facility for people diagnosed with chronic mental illness in a residential neighborhood. In this scenario students are encouraged to locate varying positions from the standpoints of people who occupy different roles in a community (e.g., elderly people in the neighborhood who have misconceptions about mental illness, parents of young children, low-income home owners, state officials, members of the National Alliance for Mental Health, or the future residents), all of whom will have particular biases, values, and interests that influence the position they take on the agency decision. This activity allows students to consider how a variety of community standpoints influences decision making and to place their own standpoints in the context of others'. As students grapple with these exercises, the influences of their own standpoints on the positions they take and the fit these have with their values become more transparent and recognizable. Further, when these standpoints are explicitly articulated, students can explore their effects on clients and dialogue regarding how to mitigate any negative ramifications they identify.

These sample exercises serve to integrate the thematic material relating to diagnosis and context, critical thinking and theory, and influence of standpoint with the processes of dialogic critique in exploration of our practice approaches. As such they pose a potential method to assist students in exploring real-life practice alternatives, as well as the disconnects between contemporary mental health practice environments and the larger ideal of critical, contextual practice that embraces social work's classic justice-oriented, person-in-environment focus.

CONCLUSION

This article has explored a number of problematic issues that US social work practitioners face in the current mental health system and the accompanying conundrums that face their educators. The reader will note that the pedagogical efforts are not designed to resolve the issues for students as they transition into the world of community mental health practice. Rather, they are designed to raise respectful questions regarding the path of social work practice in the mental health world and to explore potential responses to them. These questions are also likely to trouble students and practitioners as they don't point to neat answers. The authors believe the legacy of the profession is to engage in such examinations of purposes and methods, even when they reflect ambiguity, as educators continue to keep professional commitments rich and alive through ongoing critique and dialogue in the postmodern era.

REFERENCES

American Psychiatric Association (2000). *Diagnostic and statistical manual of mental disorders, Text Revision* (4th ed.). Washington D.C.: American Psychiatric Association.
Bentley, K.J., & Taylor, M.F. (2002). A context and vision for excellence in social work practice in contemporary mental health settings. In K.J. Bentley, *Social work practice*

in mental health: Contemporary roles, tasks, and techniques (pp. 1–17). Pacific Grove, CA: Brooks/Cole.

Compton, B.R., & Galaway, B. (1999). *Social work processes* (6th ed.). Pacific Grove, CA: Brooks/Cole.

Davis, K. (2001). The intersection of fee-for-service, managed health care, and cultural competence: Implications for national health care policy and services to people of color. In N.W. Veeder & W. Peebles-Wilkins (Eds.), *Managed care services: Policy, programs, and research* (pp. 50–73). New York: Oxford University Press.

Dewees, M.P. (2002). Contested landscape: The role of critical dialog for social workers in mental health practice. *Journal of Progressive Human Services, 13*, 1, 73–83.

Gondolf, E. W. (1998). *Assessing woman battering in mental health services.* Thousand Oaks, CA.: Sage.

Hartman, A. (1994). In search of subjugated knowledge. In A. Hartman, *Reflections & controversy.* Washington, D.C.: NASW Press.

Healy, L.M. (2001). *International social work.* New York: Oxford University Press.

Hepworth, D.H., Rooney, R.H., & Larsen, J. (2001). *Direct social work practice: Theory and skills* (6th ed.). Pacific Grove, CA: Brooks/Cole.

Hoff, M.D., Huff, D.D. & Ord, L.M. (1996). The social worker's ethical obligations to society: An assessment of charity and justice contributions of social workers. *Arete, 21*(1), 47–60.

Kirk, S.A., & Kutchins, H. (1992). *The selling of DSM: The rhetoric of science in psychiatry.* New York: Aldine de Gruyter.

Kirk, S.A., & Kutchins, H. (1994). The myth of the reliability of DSM. *The Journal of Mind and Behavior, 15*, 1–2.

Kirst-Ashman, K.K. & Hull, G.H. (2002). *Understanding generalist practice.* Pacific Grove, CA: Brooks/Cole.

Kutchins, H., & Kirk, S.A., (1988). The business of diagnosis: *DSM-III* and clinical social work. *Social Work, 33*, 215–220.

Kutchins, H., & Kirk, S.A., (1995). Should DSM be the basis for teaching social work practice in mental health? No! *Journal of Social Work Education, 31*, 159–165.

Kutchins, H. & Kirk, S.A. (1997). *Making us crazy: DSM: The psychiatric bible and the creation of mental disorders.* New York: Free Press.

Jackson, V. (2002). In our own voice: African-American stories of oppression, survival, and recovery in mental health systems. *The International Journal of Narrative Therapy and Community, 2*, 11–31.

Lacasse, J.R., & Gomory, T. (2003). Is graduate social work education promoting a critical approach to mental health practice? *Journal of Social Work Education, 39*, 3, 383–408.

Lieberman, A. (1998). *The social workout book.* Thousand Oaks, CA: Pine Forge Press.

Midgley, J. (1995). *Social development: The developmental perspective in social welfare.* Thousand Oaks, CA: Sage Publications.

Midgley, J. (1999). Social development in social work: Learning from global dialogue. In C.S. Ramanathan & R.J. Link (Eds.), *All our futures: Principles and resources for social work practice in a global era* (pp. 193–205). Belmont, CA: Brooks/Cole.

Miller, K.E., Worthington, G.J., Muzurovic, J., Tipping, S., & Goodman, A. (2002). Bosnian refugee and the stressor of exile: A narrative study. *American Journal of Orthopsychiatry, 72*, 341–354.

Pheterson, G. (1990). Alliances between Women: Overcoming internalized oppression and internalized domination. In L. Albrecht & R.M. Brewer (Eds.), *Bridges of power: Women's multicultural alliances*, (pp. 34–48). Philadelphia: New Society Publishers.

Roche, S.E., (2004). Social Work with Children and Families II Course Syllabus, University of Vermont (unpublished).

Rowe, W., Hanley, J., Moreno, E.R., & Mould, J. (2000). Voices of social work practice: International reflections on the effects of globalization. Social Work and Globalization (Special Issue). *Canadian Social Work, 2*, 1, 65–86.

Sands, R.S. (2001). *Clinical social work practice in behavioral mental health: A postmodern approach to practice with adults*. Boston: Allyn & Bacon.

Specht, H. & Courtney, M. (1994). *Unfaithful angels: How social work has abandoned its mission*. New York: Free Press.

Spitzer, R.L., Gibbon, M., Skodol, A.E., & First, M.B. (Eds.) (1994). *DSM-IV Case Book*. Washington, D.C.: American Psychiatric Association.

Warshaw, C. (2003). Creating systems change: Addressing domestic violence, trauma & mental health policy issues. Chicago: Domestic Violence & Mental Health Policy Initiative (unpublished).

Warshaw, C., Moroney, G., & Barnes, H. (2003). Report on Mental health issues & service need in the Chicago Area Domestic Violence Advocacy programs. Chicago: Domestic Violence & Mental Health Policy Initiative (unpublished).

Watters, C. (2001). Emerging paradigms in the mental health care of refugees. *Social Science & Medicine, 52*, 1709–1718.

Weick, A. (1999). Guilty knowledge. *Families in Society, 80*, 4, 327–332.

Williams, J.B., & Spitzer, R.L. (1995). Should the DSM be the basis for teaching social work practice in mental health? Yes! *Journal of Social Work Education, 31*, 148–153.

Ethnopsychiatric Approach to Immigration and Mental Health

Marie-Rosaire Kalanga Wa Tshisekedi, MSW

IMMIGRATION

Current technology and globalization have led to increased cooperation between different countries and in various areas: social, demographic, political, cultural, and economic. This very common phenomenon of the modern world results in a particular dynamic among populations that emigrate and immigrate. This necessitates adaptation and integration into a new environment with very contrasted values, often diametrically opposed to those of the society of origin. Gauthier et al. (1985) describe immigration as the "entry into a country of non-native persons" [translation] (*Robert* French dictionary) or "the establishment of strangers in a country" [translation] (*Quillet* French dictionary) (p. 3). Thus, immigrants, who are strangers in the host country and have a different culture than native persons, naturally have a different way of doing things and expressing themselves.

Immigration, whether by choice or constrained, is invariably a source of stress. Immigrants experience emotions and physical manifestations from the time of departure from their country of origin to the moment they adapt to their new environment. When additional factors are added to the stress provoked by migration (unemployment, poor knowledge of the language in the resettlement country, nonrecognition of diplomas, separation from family, etc.), mental health becomes increasingly vulnerable. When the immigration is accompanied by apprehension, integration itself can be a source of helplessness and lead to both mental and physical problems.

The immigrants' new physical environment subjects them to various influences, compelling them to experience changes that are not always desired, which in turn can impact their emotional state during adaptation and integration. Immigrants thus face a difficult situation that seems to require more effort than is possible in order to remain in a state of balance. Anxiety symptoms such as unexplained fears, permanent worry, nervousness, and tension can also surface. Self-esteem is often affected when someone feels devalued and is made to feel worthless. This erosion of self-esteem is compounded by feelings of guilt at being in such a situation. These symptoms may appear on the physiological level in the form of insomnia, loss of appetite, or a tendency to depression, aspects that can affect health. According to the World Health Organization (WHO), health is defined as "a state of physical, psychological and social well-being" [translation] (Postel, 1995). In Canada, the concept of health translates to the happiness of a person who is in control of his life and who feels both that he is valued and a productive member of his society.

MENTAL HEALTH

Mental health "does not arise from a lack of problems but rather from the ability to resolve them when they arise. As well as promoting self-esteem, this ability brings about a true inner well being" (Desmarais et al., 2000, p. 3). The Comité de la santé mentale du Québec[1] (CSMQ) defines mental health according to several factors, including: biology, which takes into account genetic components; psychodevelopmental aspects, which emphasize emotional components; and contextual factors, which take into account the integration of a person into his environment while considering his relations to others. According to Desmarais et al. (2000), the concept of mental health takes into account the significance of harmony, of social and psychological integration, of quality of life and overall well being. It also considers personal fulfillment and self-actualization, personal adaptation and the reciprocal influences of the individual, the group and the environment.

Sutter (cited by Postel, 1995, p. 48) defines mental health as an "ability of the psyche to function in a harmonious, pleasant and efficient way, and to be flexible in the face of difficult situations while being able to regain a state of balance" [translation]. Thus the concept of adaptation plays an important role in mental well being. Mental health implies living in harmony with the environment, being able to solve both internal and external problems and being able to deal with inevitable frustrations. The inability to accomplish this precludes good mental health as the risk exists of externalizing doubts and unresolved conflicts through a neurosis, or possibly decompensate, losing touch with reality, and even developing psychosis. It is a well-known fact that moving to a new country and culture inevitably leads to stress without necessarily affecting mental health. However, mental health becomes endangered when other risk factors are compounded with the stress of migration (Beiser, 1988).

The migratory experience is a life project that involves a certain trajectory and includes many stages that cannot be avoided. A specific dynamic is experienced, ranging from the subjective to the objective, from the emotional to the rational, from the imaginary to the reality. As stated by Fronteau, "Our actions (thoughts, behaviours, words) are responses based on our influences, either internal (emotions, desires, fears), or external (situations, conditions, circumstances). Everything is a question of attitude, a pendulum between a certain psychological disposition (internal) and behavior (external)" [translation] (Fronteau in Legault, 2000, p. 2).

Period Prior to Departure: Premigratory Context

The concept of premigratory context refers to the conditions of departure and the mental state of a person who has decided to leave the country of origin to live elsewhere for various reasons. These conditions vary according to whether the immigrant has chosen to leave his country or is compelled by situation and difficult circumstances. In both cases, stress related to departure from the country of origin is experienced. This stress is imputed to the immigrant's ambivalence, which may be related to the choice of leaving the country, leaving personal possessions in the hope of attaining better ones or instead remaining in the country, choosing the propitious moment for departure, choosing who will leave (alone, in a couple, with family), the anticipated length of the stay (short, long or undetermined); all these elements provide clues as to the state of the immigrant prior to departure.

The experience is somewhat different for refugees. The premigratory stress situation is exacerbated as departure is made in tragic circumstances of flight, with little preparation, which has consequences upon arrival in the resettlement country. In the face of the mourning process that arises from separation with those left behind (spouse, children or one of the children), the full extent of the psychological drama unfolds.

Period During the Stay: Postmigratory Context

The postmigratory context refers to the immigrant's experiences once in the resettlement country. This includes a wide range of losses that the migrant must face in the new environment. Life must be rebuilt at all levels: social, relational, occupational, cultural, institutional, environmental, linguistic, etc.

The various processes that newly arrived immigrants face during inser-tion into the new society include acculturation, a process of cultural change (Legault, 2000). Abou refers to it as a concept that includes "all cultural interferences that immigrants and their children experience at all levels of adaptation and integration, resulting from constant conflict between their own culture and that of the resettlement culture" [transla-tion] (in Legault, 2000, p. 79).

In their effort to adapt, immigrants must also deal with conflicting atti-tudes that will occasionally make insertion very difficult. These include mechanisms of exclusion that lead to diverse and sometimes surprising expression of difference, which can be divided into three categories. The goal of the first one is to neutralize the differences, i.e., stereotypes and ethnocentrism. The second is used to devaluate the difference, i.e., preju-dice, harassment and xenophobia. The third strongly exploits differences, i.e., racism and discrimination.

Another issue that immigrants face during the postmigratory phase is a lack of support from the family network on which they were dependent in the country of origin. This lack of support can lead to worry and anxiety, i.e., psychological, social, and mental disorders. According to Bernier, cultural changes are stressors that can cause psychosomatic symptoms, which are often "the tip of the iceberg. The medical consultation becomes the first place for screening psychosocial problems and mental disorders" [translation] (1993, p. 89).

APPROPRIATENESS OF MENTAL HEALTH SERVICES FOR IMMIGRANTS

The delivery of mental health care to immigrants and communities stemming from immigration often fails to take into account the cultural diversity of these communities. More often than not, according to Bibeau et al. (1992), the care plan is based on models developed for the Québec population, considered homogeneous but for its basic cultural dichotomy (French-speaking vs. English speaking). The approach prevalent in Québec tends to cluster all immigrants into a homogeneous group whose cultural characteristics are taken into account only in an unrealistic fash-ion, and this approach too simply overlays demographic, economic, social, and contextual variables. In other words, a uniform approach is applied more or less in a similar fashion to all situations. However, cultural communities already possess their own approach to health and illness, which includes knowledge of the body and its functioning, under-standing of the person and the various components, a know-how com-posed of reactions and responses to problems, as well as a way of being that is consistent with the values of the group with regard to life and humankind. Helping these communities can be most efficiently achieved when attention is put on their mode of communication and their percep-tion of the new environment.

According to Gravel (1993), Montréal establishments are ill-equipped to provide health services to immigrant populations, which often go beyond the issue of physical or linguistic accessibility. Despite the little attention it afforded ethnic communities, the Commission Rochon has recognized that services are poorly adapted to current Québec society and that systemic discrimination and racist stereotypes are indeed present within the social services aimed at new immigrants. In a research report presented to the Commission, Bibeau (1987) pro-poses a style of intervention in tune with culturally related issues, taking into account "culturally necessary" needs, i.e., an approach specifically relevant to the immigrant situation and responsive to the basic social and physical needs demonstrated at the time of evaluation. He also suggests that all caregivers learn to approach problems while taking into account the cultural slant.

Health professionals (psychiatrists, psychologists, nurses, and social workers) consider that immigrants, who are still closely attached to their culture, present particular challenges in mental health intervention. Their feelings of helplessness and the lack of resources or available tools for efficient intervention stem from language and cultural issues. To bridge the gap resulting from these challenges and attempt to better help these populations, efforts have been made by various caregivers to try and define the modalities of better access to health and social services for eth-nic communities. A new approach has been developed that takes into account the social characteristics of immigrants and the incompatibility of standard Western therapeutic practices with the cultural idiosyncrasies of immigrants from non-Western cultures.

The Hôpital Jean-Talon in Montréal is one of those institutions that has implemented, within its psychiatry department, a specialized program aimed at immigrants and their families facing mental health problems. This program was inspired by the model developed by Tobie Nathan (1986, 1988, 1994) in France. In 2001, the Prix d'Excellence des Hôpitaux du Québec was awarded to the hospital for this innovative approach. The Centre Jeunesse de Laval, the CLSC Saint-Michel, the

Montreal Children's Hospital, and the Hôpital Hotel-Dieu offer similar programs, which attempt to rebuild, through intervention, a community-type relationship that is found in the immigrant's root society, namely ethnopsychiatry.

ETHNOPSYCHIATRY

The etymology of the term "ethno" comes from ancient Greek meaning "nation"; by extension it signified "people," "tribes," "foreign population," etc. This term aroused curiosity and was related to "primitives" and "savages" by comparison to "White, civilized" Western man (Fourasté, 1985, p. 15).

Ethnopsychiatry has had several influences. First related to folk psychology, it then became linked to colonial psychiatry. More recently, it appears more closely connected to anthropology and ethnology. From the outset, it has promoted the inherent confirmation of ethnic disparity, creating in effect a psychiatry department reserved for "noncivilized" peoples, healed by sorcerers. Despite this trend, mental illnesses will long remain defined based on Western criteria, which fails to recognize cultural differences (Corin, 1997).

According to Laplantine (1998), Georges Devereux should be considered the true founder of ethnopsychiatry, despite the fact that Devereux himself attributes the first use of the term to the famous Haitian psychiatrist, Dr. Louis Mars, who apparently coined the term (Devereux, 1982). For Devereux, ethnopsychiatry is unique in that it allows the therapist to define "cultural normality or abnormality, the manipulations and reinterpretations that the patient operates on the cultural matter and the way in which he uses them" [translation] (Devereux, 1977, p. 105). Advances made in psychoanalytic ethnopsychiatry are owed to Devereux. He was able to bridge the gap between psychoanalysis, which underscores the universality of the unconscious, and ethnology, which takes into account the specificity of clinical profiles evidenced by cultural diversity (Paquette, 1999).

The goal of ethnopsychiatry is to link four types of discourse: the first is composed of narrations provided by ethnologists; the second is based on a "scholarly," i.e., psychiatric, discourse; the third examines the psychological dimension of societies; and the fourth represents the synthesis of the above discourses. This ethnopsychiatric discourse is personal and unique to each ethnopsychiatrist.

Ethnopsychiatry attempts to understand an individual's way of being when placed within a given context. It strives to understand how he comprehends, appreciates or explains things, events and facts that come from within or from his environment. It involves a discovery of the psychic characteristics and inconsistencies that come about in the traditional environment (Fourasté, 1985).

According to Tousignant and Murphy, ethnopsychiatry is defined as "the study of the relationship between behaviour, therapeutic services and the culture of origin of the patient and the therapist" [translation] (1978, p. 321).

For Nathan (1994), ethnopsychiatry relates both to the cultural description of mental disorder and the analysis of individual psychic functioning. It incorporates the principles of the analytical approach, and takes into account other aspects (cultural or traditional) and more specifically attempts to find therapeutic responses adapted to patients whose knowledge and ways of doing things contrast with the discourse of Western psychotherapy.

TRANSCULTURAL PSYCHIATRY

The field of transcultural psychiatry has expanded in the United States and Canada, particularly at McGill University in Montréal where it came about in 1956, owing to the work of physicians Wittkower, Murphy and Prince (Marchand, 2000). These researchers specifically investigated the prevalence of mental disorders, the observation of ethnic differences on a behavioural level, the variability of mental contents and the occurrence of syndromes specific to the cultural context (Corin et al., 1987).

Transcultural psychiatry in North America has been dominated by theoretical research, while in France the emphasis has been on the works of caregivers confronted with the real situation of patients from other cultures. Although the French share the interest of North American researchers of the impact of culture and personal experience, they differ in their focus on the psychoanalytic approach (Corin, 1997).

According to Devereux, the term "transcultural" is applied to psychiatry by psychiatrists or anthropologists. Used in this manner, it refers to what he calls crosscultural psychiatry. In his opinion, transcultural psychiatry, in the meaning of those who have misappropriated the term, requires an "in-depth knowledge of the culture of the ill person" [translation] (Corin, 1997). Thus, this approach to psychiatry requires that the culture of each patient must be thoroughly understood. Based on his experiences (psychiatric hospitals, teaching of psychoanalytical ethnopsychiatry and practice of psychoanalysis), he finds it somewhat absurd to require that psychiatrists possess a detailed knowledge of the culture of each patient or an expert knowledge of all cultures.

Devereux abandoned the term "transcultural" and condemned its "incorrect misappropriation" [translation] (Devereux, 1982, p. 18) choosing rather the term "metacultural" to emphasize all that lies beyond culture. In his opinion, the crucial aspect is to understand the function of culture itself and the nature of the universal culture pattern from which each culture is a variation. He emphasized the need for a general knowledge of culture theory by underlining the relationship between culture and mental health (which are interrelated). Culture as a real experience relates to "a manner in which the individual lives and experiences culture in a state of mental health or psychological disorder" [translation] (Devereux, 1977, p. 81).

According to Devereux, transcultural psychiatry is the study of the "relationship between culture proper and any other and all other psychopathology. It is thus opposed to cross-cultural psychiatry and psychotherapy" [translation]. To this, he adds that, in a way, the term transcultural itself points to the lack of precision of the field of ethnopsychiatry in general (Devereux, 1982).

After Devereux, Nathan in France (1988) was the first to modify the therapeutic framework. He points out the difficulties inherent to providing therapeutic care to patients from non-Western cultures. He then developed a model of ethnopsychiatric consultation aimed at offering true psycholanalysis-based psychotherapy to those who present symptoms in deeply "culturally encoded" terms, to avoid too brief psychiatric care, hospitalizations and an exaggerated use of psychotropic medication. A first ethnopsychiatric consultation in France took place in 1979 at the Hôpital d'Avicenne at Bobigny. The immigrant patients, mostly from North Africa, Africa and the Caribbean are mostly described in terms of deficiencies (fantasmatic, elaborative, social). Clinical ethnopsychiatry arose from the transformation of these presumed deficiencies into sources of enrichment and new therapeutic techniques (Nathan, 1988).

THE ETHNOPSYCHIATRIC APPROACH

The originality of the ethnopsychiatric approach developed by Nathan has generated much interest and attention. The innovative aspect resides in the therapeutic device of the clinical approach. It is a model inspired by "traditional" societies where the group itself serves as a means to solve problems.

As underlined by Gratton (2000), ethnopsychiatry is not only a way that takes into accounts the relations between individuals but it is also a transitional approach. Interested in the cultural encoding of psychic functioning, it is based on the elaboration of the experience of the crisis caused by a loss of cultural buffers and the difficulty of transition to another cultural universe (Ondogh-Essalt, 1998).

METHODOLOGICAL PRINCIPLE IN ETHNOPSYCHIATRY: COMPLEMENTARISM

Devereux termed this multidisciplinary approach "complementarism," a basic tenet of ethnopsychiatry. It is defined as the "possibility of completely understanding a phenomenon in at least two ways (complementary) that demonstrate, on one hand, that the phenomenon is both real and explainable, and on the other that each of these explanations is" whole "(and thus valid) within its own frame of reference" [translation] (Devereux, 1985, p. 13). The main point is the definition of the relationship between these various explanations. For this reason, complementarism as proposed by Devereux involves a systematic generalization that brings together all acceptable reasoning and hypothesis of the relationships between psychoanalysis, ethnology and history. In his opinion, every person, regardless of ethnic background, "functions as creator, creature, manipulator and mediator of culture in any context and in the same manner" [translation] (Devereux, 1977, p. XXII). However, he points out that ethnopsychiatry proceeds from the general (collective) to the particular (individual) and inversely, and is based on a systematic comprehension of diversified or invariable terms, similar or not, which have to be deciphered without neglecting the underlying main idea. He indicates that this double discourse is never expressed simultaneously despite complementarity. The raw facts are based on at least two discourses that complete each other but cannot be held simultaneously. Within this perspective, ethnopsychiatry assumes mastery of two distinct discourses, one linked to psychoanalysis, the other to culture. It explores the limits of both meanings, without ever trying to interpret or explain one discourse in terms of the other (Corin, 1997). Thus, psychoanalysis can reveal an aspect of the psychic life of a person in a given culture or in a given situation, without leading to a complete understanding of the process entered into by the unconscious. The mechanism of complementarity between culture and psychoanalysis has been defined by Anzieu and Nathan as "doublets" or "homologous" structures containing the same basic elements governed by similar mechanisms (in Corin, 1997).

TECHNICAL FRAMEWORK IN ETHNOPSYCHIATRY

In ethnopsychiatry, the technical framework refers to the device whose temporal and spatial structures are represented by a team of therapists, which serves several therapeutic functions and is consistent with the assumptions that guide ethnopsychiatry. This approach serves as the backdrop for the interactions that occur in the group, placed in a circle, aimed at facilitating discussion.

Thus, the practice of ethnopsychiatry involves the implementation of a team that can help better clarify the cultural information from the patient's community of origin as well as information from his or her psychic universe. This team provides context for multiple representations of "otherness." It allows for the development of a discourse that does not freeze the patient in a static representation. It assumes a function of cultural localization (through the use of the native language and evocation of traditional etiologies) and a psychological function (through the support of the team). It acts as support to the relationship among the team members by allowing the traditional etiologies to unravel all the way to evocations of the patient's deepest inner life. It serves as a go-between, a "mixed" framework, facilitating the expression of emotions. By assuming these various roles, the team device also furthers the principles underlying ethnopsychiatry.

For Moro (1993), the team therapeutic device requires an analysis of the cultural countertransference of the therapists, which can parcel out that belonging to the identity of the therapist, his professional identity, his social identity and his cultural identity. Thus, the group intervention provides additional clues helping to confirm the psychocultural diagnosis of a given behaviour. From what they perceive and hear, the therapists focus their attention on their fantasies and their emotions, which enhances their connection to the group (Mesmin, 2000).

According to the Western model of ethnopsychiatry, the role of the principal therapist is to promote discussion among members of the group, inviting the cotherapists to talk to the patient through him (See figure in

Appendix 1: Team Therapeutic Device). The cotherapists' interventions are aimed at bringing elements of clarification and comprehension to decipher the patient's discourse, given their knowledge of a wide range of cultural references and clinical expertise. According to Nathan et al. (1998), the principal therapist consults them and relies on them while reserving the right to reiterate some of their interventions and to communicate them to the patient. He must thus operate a decentration of his thoughts and his being, while mastering the general process he is initiating (Moro, 1993). Ondongh-Essalt (1994, p. 165) describes him as a person who "must have broad ethnological, psychiatric and psychopathological knowledge as well as proven clinical expertise" [translation].

The culture broker is also known as an ethnoclinical broker. His role is to elucidate the conflicts produced by the confrontation of theories from two different universes. According to Pierzo and Legault (in Legault, 2000), the cultural broker translates the patient's cultural environment, gives access to the myths, proverbs, metaphors, non-verbal messages and paralanguage. The group depends on him to understand the subtleties of the spoken language and decode and demystify certain cultural behaviours. He acts as a support for all, as he clarifies formulations that the patient or therapists have trouble understanding. He holds a double knowledge, that of the patient's culture and that of the host society. He helps to understand certain subtle behaviours, laden with information, and to identify the disorders experienced by the patient, and can suggest leads to help the caregivers as well as the patients. As underscored by Nathan and Lewertowski (1998), neutrality has no place; on the contrary he must sometimes know how to stir up conflict to disengage the patient from a double constraint.

The team also calls on an interpreter when patients have difficulty understanding the language spoken by the therapists. His role is to establish a bridge between patients and caregivers, with whom he does not share the language or the culture. The interpreter removes the obstacle of language by translating and transmitting the message, and also by enabling an exchange that facilitates communication. This role differs from the cultural broker, among other things, in the sense that he goes beyond the words themselves by avoiding lags in meaning that can result in different understanding of the facts. According to Salmi (1986), the presence of a cultural broker or an interpreter is essential to understanding what the patient feels. Indeed, the patient's images are linked to an inner cultural process and can only be unraveled in the patient's native language. Thus the associations of the illness translate themselves better in the patient's language, because in all societies, symptoms are linked to the difficulties inherent in communicating with others.

TOOLS OF THE TRADE IN ETHNOPSYCHIATRY

Traditional etiologies

Traditional etiologies serve as working tools for the spoken language and have a restructuring function. The meaning or meanings that are attributed to a given fact or event, can also explain what we have done to create our problems or to protect ourselves from them (Corin et al., 1987). These etiologies are based on logic from traditional therapies, of thought processes that attribute a specific value or meaning to the problems. The evocations that arise lead to action in the minds of the patient and therapist. For example, one can suffer from anemia after having been eaten by one's aunt (sorcery), after having been inhabited by one's grandfather (possession), etc. These etiologies can be objects, concepts, metaphors, traditional medicines, interpretations, narratives, proverbs, customs, or myths. Their role is to help the person understand the symptoms, to give them meaning, to understand their roots, to gain specific knowledge, to adopt a position toward the symptoms and its roots and decide on a course of action. Patients refer to these etiologies to give meaning to their illness or difficulties. Traditional etiologies encode the symptoms. They provide a framework amenable to discussion, acknowledge the legitimacy of cultural interpretations, and free the discourse of the patients and their families. Furthermore, traditional etiologies allow for a series of associations that recast the symptoms in the personal and collective "history" of the patients (Corin, 1997) and can initiate a process of elaboration. According to Nathan (1988), these etiologies are processes or technical operators that result in a complex relational dynamic. They can also be considered as levers (cultural and /or therapeutic) as long as they facilitate the insight of the patient or therapist. In addition, Devereux (cited in Corin, 1997) regards myths as impersonal "cold chambers" where persons store their fantasies. Ethnopsychiatrists must manipulate them in order for these fantasies to emerge.

Modern etiologies

Modern etiologies refer to explanations of a person's psychic functioning based on the Freudian concept of the unconscious. They help to better understand the intrapsychic dynamic and eventually to formulate hypotheses.

These are the basis of Western psychotherapies. For example, the dream is the "royal road" to the unconscious; they can also be referred to as defense mechanisms such as repression, transference, counter-transference, etc.

Semantic Bombardment

Semantic bombardment is an active process of the grasp of the patient's problem through the lens of several cultures. It is the elaboration of a fragment of the patient's problem to offer him a different outlook and understanding of his experiences while respecting the limits inherent to the understanding of his culture. When the elaboration process is initiated, it results in the deconstruction of the discourder the patient wishes to present. At the end of the process, the patient is presented with a reorganized set of his own elements through the work of the team of therapists (Nathan, 1988). For Nathan, the feeling of mastering psychoanalytic knowledge enables the caregivers to bring external support to the patient, by reiterating the identifications or simply letting him reach them intuitively (Nathan, 1988). Semantic bombardment is the use of these etiologies during the therapeutic process. It produces a "rupture in the patient's discourse of what is perceived and felt" [translation] (Moro, 1993, p. 272).

CONCLUSION

Immigrant populations are changing the profile of the host society through attempts to integrate and adapt while respecting the respective cultures and values. As every culture evolves through contact with other cultures, immigrants and natives of the host country mutually influence each other. They act as "cultural yeasts" (Devereux, 1977, p. 76) and attempt to find adequate means of getting closer while avoiding conflicts. Efforts are being made in mental health to implement services that take into account the culture of immigrants.

The therapeutic perspective of the ethnopsychiatric approach is based on three essential principles that act as a bridge linking all participants in the host society, including those in various hospital settings, rehabilitation centers, schools, and community organizations.

For Immigrants

The ethnopsychiatric approach gives immigrants the chance to express deep inner thoughts and impersonal notions stemming from their culture.

Immigrants provide the expression of experiences that are specific to them and provide a window into a family, cultural, or occupational past. This expression brings a new dimension, an unknown aspect that can help resolve verbal or behavioral inconsistencies and facilitate understanding of certain actions. For example, an immigrant father finds unjust and incomprehensible that "corporal punishment" administered to his child could lead him to the court system in the host society, as it is only perceived as an act of education.

The difficulties are also great for certain immigrants who have secretly left their country in the hope of escaping the evil eye, sorcery, or any other occult act deemed malevolent. This also applies to those who converted to a more lax religion or who have chosen to distance themselves from certain traditional practices, and who now have to address these within the framework of ethnopsychiatry. For them, this can only seem confusing, paradoxical, and a source of doubt. The source of this unease, this doubt, and this paradox lies in the cultural history of each, akin to a trademark, sometimes indelible, that one carries within and which cannot be swiftly erased in the name of integration, assimilation, or conversion. The memory of culture, even when repressed, always leads certain cultural elements to resurface through various cues in everyday life and particularly when all seems to go wrong. It is a fact that every culture has established mechanisms to meet certain expectations or resolve certain problems in an appropriate manner that meets the cultural norms. For example, a Catholic person might refer to the "Holy Name of Jesus," the Pentecostal to the "Blood of Jesus," the Muslim to the "Name of Allah," the animist to the "spirit of the elders," etc.

For Caregivers

The cultural description, baring the patient's problematic situation, promotes a process of intervention through the ethnopsychiatric approach using a preliminary mini-inventory (See Appendix 2). It provides new leads, exhibits up-to-date knowledge and forms a new interpretation of the situation that requires intervention and a mastery of the implemented technique. It thus warrants taking into account the cultural dimension integral to each person.

The integration of this approach via various theoretical concepts helps to elucidate the cultural discourse and evaluate the optimal moment to adopt the ethnopsychiatric approach whose pertinence lends itself to a very practical application and to active participation in the therapeutic team. The ethnopsychiatric approach, contrary to many other approaches, is an additional tool enabling caregivers to consider various paths to understanding and treating mental illness while addressing the cultural dimensions, and keeping in mind that the "touchstone of mental health is not adaptation in itself, but the capacity of the patient to undergo successive readaptations, without losing the feeling of this own continuity in time" [translation] (Devereux, 1977, p. 75)

For Institutions

Occasionally, the presence of cultural elements in the patient's or families' understanding of their problems make it difficult to administer medical care and provide appropriate intervention. The ethnopsychiatric approach enables patients and caregivers to get a new outlook on the difficulties. It affords patients and caregivers to adopt a "new" dialogue based on the cultural and social reality of patients, and offers new directions for treatment. The mere fact of introducing a new approach in an institution as hierarchized as a hospital setting shows an open attitude toward the immigrant population. This attitude should be encouraged to ensure the implementation of this approach in settings other than hospitals, and thus transcend institutional environments.

The appreciation of this new approach must be a process that is not limited to the creation of a cultural narrative, but also one that integrates it, in a harmonious way, within the body of knowledge in methods of analysis and models of therapeutic interventions. Combining the ethnopsychiatric approach with already known and established approaches could lead to more effective ways of conducting research aimed at better serving immigrant populations. The ethnopsychiatric approach is often a last recourse for the patient, who has previously made several attempts to solve his or her problems, and for the caregivers who now feel inadequate in the face of "another" reality that they cannot completely understand. This approach serves as an additional element of understanding in the causes of the problems as well as their treatment.

It should however be noted that ethnopsychiatry is not adapted to all and also has contraindications, particularly when a pathology manifests itself with obvious symptoms. First and foremost the goal will be to alleviate the symptoms despite the presence of potential cultural elements in the patient's discourse. It should be noted that the application of the ethnopsychiatric approach often is confronted with very strong resistance, which can be overcome only if we possess proficiency in the art of dialogue, as the application of the ethnopsychiatric approach is an art, the art of discussion to understand the root of the problem through the lens of the family or the patient, while being able to manipulate psychoanalytic and anthropological concepts. Community organizations serving families could implement a "transcultural mediation" service based on ethnopsychiatric principles.

NOTE

1. The CSMQ acts as an advisory committee for the Ministre de la Santé et des Services Sociaux du Québec that contributes to decisions made in the field of mental health.

BIBLIOGRAPHY

American Psychiatric Association. (1996). *DSM-IV. Manuel Diagnostique et statistique des troubles mentaux.* (4th ed.). Paris: Masson.

Ami-Quebec et al. (1993). *La maladie mentale. Un guide régional destiné aux familles.* (2nd ed.). Montréal:

Beiser, M. et al. (1988). *Puis ... la porte s'est ouverte: Probléme de santé mentale des immigrants et des refugies.* Canada: Santé et bien-être social.

Bernier, D. (1993). Le stress des réfugiés et ses implications pour la pratique et la formation. *Service social, 42* (1).

Bibeau, G. et al. (1992). *La santé mentale et ses visages.* Montréal. Gaëtan Morin.

Corin, E. et al. (1987). *Regards anthropologiques en psychiatrie.* Montreal: Girame.

Corin. E. (1997). Playing with Limits: Nathan's Evolving Paradigm in Ethnopsychiatry in *Transcultural Psychiatry. 34*(3), 345–358.

Conseil Économique du Canada. (1991). *Le nouveau visage du Canada.* Gouvernement fédéral: Rapport synthése.

Desmarais, D. et al. (2000). *Détresse psychologique et insertion sociale des jeunes adultes.* Montréal: Les publications du Québec.

Devereux. G. (1977). *Essais d'ethnopsychiatrie générale.* (3rd ed.). Paris: Gallimard.

Devereux. G. (1982). *Psychothérapie d'un Indien des plaines.* Paris: Jean-Cyrille Godefroy.

Devereux, G. (1985). *Ethnopsychanalyse complémentariste.* Paris: Flammarion.

Fourasté. R. (1985). *Introduction à l'ethnopsychiatrie.* Toulouse: Privat.

Gauthier et al. (1985). Migrants: Trajets et trajectoires. *Revue internationale d'action communautaire, 14/15,* automne, 85.

Gratton, D. (2000). L'expertise psychologique et les familles de migrants. *Le magazine des psychologues du Québec, 17*(5), 19–21.

Gravel, S. (1992–1993). Un exemple de la contribution de l'anthropologie à la planification d'un programme de périnatalité en milieu multiculturel. *Santé Culture Health, IX* (1), 139.

Laplantine. F. (1988). *L'ethnopsychiatrie.* Paris: PUF.

Larousse. (1999). *Grand dictionnaire de la psychologie.* Paris: Bordas.

Legault, G. (2000). *L'intervention interculturelle.* Montréal: Gaëtan Morin.

Marcachand. D. (2000). Transcultural Psychiatry Une revue au confluent des cultures, *Prisme*, octobre 2000.

Mesmin, C. (2000). Le groupe thérapeutique au sein du dispositif ethnopsychiatrique. http://www.ethnopsychiatrie.net/act/Mesmin.htm

Ministère de la Sante et des Services Sociaux. (1988). *Commission d'enquête sur les services de santé et les services sociaux.* Québec: Sous la présidence de Jean Rochon.

Ministère de la Santé et des Services Sociaux. (1997). *Défi de la configuration des services de santé mantale. Pour une réponse efficace et efficient aux besoins des personnes atteintes de troubles mentaux graves.* Québec: Comité de la santé mentale du Québec.

Moro, M-R. (1992). Principes théoriques et méthodologiques de l' ethnopsychiatrie. *Santé mentale au Québec, XVII*(2) 71–98.

Moro, M-R. (1993). Principes théoriques et cliniques de l'ethnopsychiatrie. Quelques données actuelles, dans L'évolution psychiatrique. Tome 58. Fasciculel. Mars.

Moro, M-R. (2002). Enfants d'ici venus d'ailleurs. *Naître et grandir en France.* Paris: La Découverte.

Nathan, T. (1986). La folies des autres. Traité d' ethnopsychiatrie clinique. Paris: Dunod.

Nathan, T. (1988). Le sperme du diable: Paris. PUF.

Nathan, T. (1988). Psychanalyse païenne. Essais ethnopsychanalytiques. Paris: Dunod.

Nathan. T. (1993). Fier de n'avoir ni pays ni amis, quelle sottise c'était. Paris: La pensée sauvage.

Nathan, T., & Stengers, I. (1995). Médecin et sorciers. Paris: Synthélabo.

Nathan, T., & Lewertowski, C. (1998). Soigner. Le virus et le fétiche. Paris: Odile Jacob.

Nathan, T. et al (1998). Psychothérapies. Paris: Odile Jacob.

Ondongh-Essalt, E. (1994). Ethnopsychiatrie et travail social. Éléments cliniques et socio-anthropologiques pour un interpartenariat efficace des familles, dans Lien social et Politique. *RIAC, 32*, 163–178.

Ondongh-Essalt, E. (1998). Corps malade et trace de l'exil. *Revue internationale d'études Transculturelle et d'Ethnopsychanalyse clinique 1*, 75–90.

Ordre Professionnel des Travailleurs Sociaux du Quebec, (OPTSQ) (1999). Guide pour la Pratique professionnelle des travailleurs sociaux exercant en milieu hospitalier. Québec: OPTSQ.

Paquette, D. (1999). L'ethnopsychiatrie: Histoire, courant et enjeux. *Revue internationale d'études Transculturelle et d'Ethnopsychanalyse clinique, 3/4*, 158–172.

Postel, J. (1995). Dictionnaire de psychiatrie et de psychopathologie clinique. Paris: Larousse Bordas.

Salmi, H. (1986). L'interpréte, l'immigré, la langue, le langage, le corps et autres situations. In Regard sur l'immigration au quotidien en Île de France. Paris: Publication inter services migrants.

Toussignant, M., & Murphy, H.B.M. (1978). Fondements anthropologiques de l'ethnopsychiatrie. *Encycl. Méde. Chir., Paris, psychiatrie*, 4- 1978, 37715–10.

Tshisekedi, K. M-R. (2002). Santé mentale et clientéle immigrante: L' approche ethnopsychiatrique. University of Montreal: Rapport de stage pour la Maîtrise de qualification professionnelle en service social.

Viger-Rojas, C. (1999). Processus d'évaluation de l'intervention clinique du Module transculturel. Rapport-synthése. Montréal: Hôpital Jean Talon.

APPENDIX 1. SCHEMA OF INTERVENTION TEAM

Schema of Intervention Team

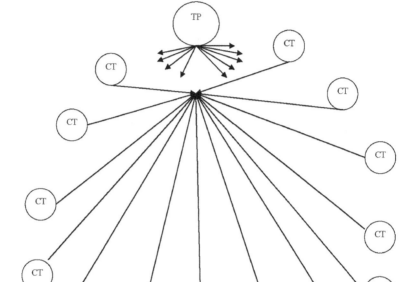

Legend:
PT = Principal therapist
CT = Co-therapists (representations of multiple "otherness")
A,B and C = Immigrant and family members
R = Referring caregiver (caregiver in charge of the file and responsible for follow-up)
M = Cultural broker or ethnoclinical broker; - I = Interpreter
Arrows indicate the direction of exchanges
Short arrows from PT to CT indicates that the pertinent interventions by the CT are integrated by the PT to further the therapeutic process.

APPENDIX 2. PRELIMINARY EVALUATION MINI-INVENTORY FOR CAREGIVERS

Brief summary of reason for consultation
Civil status
Country of origin
Reason(s) for departure (whenever possible)
Year of arrival in host country
Integration in host country
Family members in host country
Religious affiliation
Language(s) spoken and language of use

Aging and Mental Health

Neena L. Chappell, PhD, FRSC, CRC

INTRODUCTION

While physiological decline is correlated with growing older, seniors tend to suffer more from chronic than acute illness and more from functional disability than disease. Decline is also more likely with age for some diseases that affect our mental health, such as dementia. However, subjective overall well-being does not tend to decline—seniors, for example, report high perceptions of their health and of overall life satisfaction.

These facts have much relevance for practice, because our health care system is oriented toward a medical perspective and acute illness, neither of which are most appropriate for an aging society. Furthermore, mental health is still a neglected aspect when it comes to services. Seniors, like others, can and do live primarily active lives in which a health promotion approach is not only feasible but desirable. An aging society, therefore, requires a health care system that promotes health and, when disability strikes, supports rehabilitation and functioning. A health promotion perspective applies equally, irrespective of whether we are talking about physical or mental health; indeed, the two are related.

This article begins with a presentation of some health "facts" regarding aging and briefly discusses Canada's provincial and territorial health care systems. It argues for the necessity of a greater health promotion emphasis if our health care systems are to appropriately provide care for an aging society. It ends with a brief discussion of implication for practice.

SOME FACTS ABOUT AGING

Fully 83% of all seniors in Canada living at home report being diagnosed with at least one chronic health condition. The most common is arthritis and rheumatism: 39.9% of seniors suffer from this compared with 15.0% of all age groups (rising to 47.5% among those age 75+). Thirty-three percent suffer from high blood pressure; 22% have food or other allergies; 18% cataracts; 17% back problems; and 16% chronic heart problems (Statistics Canada: www.hc-sc.gc.ca/seniors, 2001). The figure for those reporting functional health problems is 18.6% among all age groups, rising to 34.2% among those 65+ and to 45.5% among those 75+ (Statistics Canada, Canadian Community Health Survey, 2000/01). Pain is a problem for many seniors, with 25% suffering chronic pain or discomfort, increasing to 37% among those age 85 years and over. Most take some form of medication, either prescription or over the counter (84%) and most (56%) are taking two or more. This figure increases to 65% among those age 85 and over (Statistics Canada, 1999; Chappell, Gee, McDonald, & Stones, 2003). That is, chronic illness characterizes old age; physical health declines as we age.

Diseases that impair cognition also increase as we age. Dementia refers to disorders with multiple cognitive deficits, the most common being Alzheimer's disease constituting approximately half of all dementias. Other types of dementia such as vascular dementia have lower prevalence. Dementia involves progressive deterioration in cognitive competence; onset is gradual and there is a continuation of symptoms. The Longitudinal Canadian Study of Health and Aging (1994) estimated the prevalence of dementia in Canada among older individuals to be 8%. Half of the individuals suffering from dementia in Canada reside in long term institutions and half within the community; two thirds are female and one third male. The prevalence increases with age. Prevalence rate for Alzheimer's disease is 5.1%.

The Canadian Study of Health and Aging also revealed risk factors for dementia: family history, low education, and head injury. Low risk is associated with suffering from arthritis and the use of nonsteroidal anti-inflammatory drugs. Symptoms of Alzheimer's disease tend to reveal a stage by stage progression: forgetfulness, then confusion, then failure to recognize familiar people, loss of memory for recent events, disorientation, and then loss of all verbal abilities (Reisberg, Ferris, deLeon, & Crook, 1982). Despite the devastating effects of dementia for those who suffer from it and for their family and loved ones, it is to be noted that at any point in time, fully 92% of Canadian seniors do not have this disease.

Furthermore, normal aging sees few significant changes in cognition. Cognition refers to thoughts and perceptions rather than feelings and volitions. It refers to the processing of information including memory, which refers to the residues of previous information processing. While 28% of seniors experience some type of memory problems, this is a complex area. Memories can refer to episodic memory, that is, memories of information processed at a particular time, and knowledge, memories integrated into composite structures not related to particular episodes.

Sensory memory (information from the environment for a very brief interval) shows limited decline with age (Craik & Jennings, 1992). Short term memory includes both primary memory (past storage) and working memory (active manipulation of information). These same authors reveal no appreciable decline until very late in life. The latter, working memory, does decline with age (Hultsch & colleagues, 1992). Long term memory also appears to change with age with older people remembering less than younger people. Older people are disadvantaged with unfamiliar information, when the material is presented at a fast rate and with tasks that require effortful rather than automatic processing. However, they are able to learn new ways of learning (Chappell et al., 2003). There seems to be more loss in recognition than in recall of information with age. There is considerable retention of very old memories into old age.

Likewise, intelligence is multidimensional and can include, for example, verbal comprehension, word fluency, number intelligence, spatial orientation, associative memory, perceptual speed, and inductive reasoning. Longitudinal research (Schaie, 1996) suggests that intelligence generally does not decline with age until very late old age. That is, there are few significant changes in memory and intelligence as we age, despite the fact that diseases such as dementia become more prevalent in old age.

While chronic conditions are more likely to occur in old age, this is not necessarily the case with mental illness. For example, major depression does not increase as we age; it is not the most prevalent among seniors. Fully 88.6% of all Canadians 12+ say they have no risk of depression; among those 65+ the figure is 92.4% (Statistics Canada, Canadian Community Health Survey, 2000/01). Depression can nevertheless be devastating for those it affects and it increases the risk of mortality from physical illness, increases the risks of suicide, contributes to cognitive decline among the nondemented elderly, and is an early manifestation of dementia. Although the prevalence of major depression appears to decline with age, there is some dispute as to whether or not there is undiagnosed depression among seniors (Gallo, Rabins & Hopkins, 1999). There are gender differences in self-reports of depression with females more likely reporting feelings of depression than males. Depression is particularly important among seniors because success rates range between 60% and 80%, meaning that the issue of undiagnosed depression becomes very important, particularly if there is a misdiagnosis, for example, of dementia, when in fact the person is suffering from depression and is treatable.

Furthermore, despite physical declines as we age, perceptions of health do not necessarily decrease. For example, seniors perceive their health to be good, very good or excellent (78%). This decreases to only 71% among those age 85 and over, where women are more likely to rate their health as only fair or poor than is true of men (Statistics Canada, 1999). That is, subjective health is more "optimistic" than objective measures might suggest.

Turning to mental health, mental well-being can be seen as the subjective evaluation of one's overall quality of life and throughout the literature is referred to as happiness, life satisfaction, morale, and trait affect. As noted by Stones and Kozma (1980), regardless of the measure, different measures of well-being are highly correlated with another. Interestingly, mental well-being (or mental health) measures show few differences either with age or with gender. That is, females do not have decreased mental well-being when compared with men, and seniors do not have decreased mental well-being compared with younger individuals. In addition, most older individuals score within the positive half range of the various indexes (Chappell et al., 2003; Myers & Diener, 1995). The consistency of these findings is evident among rich and poor as well as men and women and people of different ages.

When asking Canadians age 15 and over, in 2000/01, 27.8% rated their mental health as excellent, 39.2% very good, 26.1% good, and 6.9% fair or poor. Among those age 65+, 28.7% rated their mental health as excellent, 37.3% very good, 27.5% good and 6.5% fair or poor. In terms of life satisfaction, those 15+ reveal 32.6% saying they were very satisfied, 52.7% satisfied, 10.0% neutral, and 4.6% dissatisfied. Among those 65+ the figures were 37.5%, 51.9%, 7.1% and 3.5% respectively (Statistics Canada, Canadian Community Health Survey, 2002).

Data from the 1994 and 1995 National Population Health Survey (NPHS) reveal that in terms of a sense of coherence (a view of the world that life is meaningful, events are comprehensible, and challenges are manageable), while 28% of Canadians are high in a sense of coherence, those over age 75 are three times more likely than 18- to 19-year-olds to score high. Self-esteem and mastery improve with age, peaking in middle adulthood followed by only modest decline in the later years. That is, seniors exhibit favorable and often better psychological well-being, better mental health than do younger adults (Federal Provincial and Territorial Provincial Advisory Committee on Population Health, 1999).

In sum, we are more likely to suffer poor physical health as we age than when we were younger. Chronic conditions rather than acute diseases are more likely to afflict us in old age. We are also more likely to suffer from the cognitive disease of dementia. Importantly, mental health and well-being does not decline in the same way. Indeed, in many respects, mental health is better in old age than during younger years, despite declines in physical health and increases in disease. Taking a holistic view of health and recognizing that physical health declines but psychological well-being does not to the same extent is important for the way we approach and treat seniors when they run into difficulty with their physical health and mental health. This leads us to a discussion of current health care systems and of health care systems that might be more appropriate, that is, ones that embrace a health promotion perspective generally and a rehabilitation and functioning perspective when disability does strike. We turn now to this discussion.

CANADIAN HEALTH CARE SYSTEMS

The medical dominance of Canada's health care systems (in Canada each province has responsibility for delivery of health care to its residents), like that throughout the industrialized world, is well-established. Medicine has a monopoly to confer medical license in order to practice as a doctor and medical schools and the medical profession control the curriculum within medical schools. That is, medicine has professional autonomy and control in which physicians themselves define the scope of their work, create their own standards of practice and maintain the right to enforce those standards (Freidson, 1970). It is they who decide who can be admitted to hospital and who can receive prescription medications as well as a variety of medical tests. In some provinces such as British Columbia they control who can see a specialist. Although Canada has universal medicare for all citizens, it does not have socialized medicine; doctors work primarily on a fee-for-service basis with a guaranteed third party payer. The government and ultimately the tax payer guarantees that they will be paid for their work (Segall & Chappell, 2000).

Both the rise and maintenance of their professional dominance rests in part on their expert knowledge, which patients do not have, as well as their ability to eliminate their competition. Some competitors such as homeopaths and osteopaths were co-opted; others such as pharmacists, nurses, anesthetists, and x-ray technicians were subordinated; and others were for many years excluded from legitimate practice, such as midwives and clergy (Gritzer, 1981). Perhaps not surprisingly, physicians tend to be male and other health care workers tend to be female. Women entering the profession tend to be at the bottom of the hierarchy, that is, they are rarely heads of large prestigious services, large teaching hospitals, or medical centers. Rather, they tend to be in general practice, family practice, and primary care, where they lack the kind of occupational autonomy and power that male physicians typically posess. This has been demonstrated for England, the United States, and Norway (Elston, 1993; Riska & Weiger, 1993). Other health care workers, including social workers, are predominantly female but subordinate to physicians.

The biomedical model views disease as related to changes in specific organs of the body that are caused by pathogenic agents such as germs. Biomedical treatment, therefore, attempts to control the causes, often through drug therapy, or by removing them through surgery, or both. The medical model views disease as an objective biophysical phenomenon characterized by a change in functioning of the biological organism that is our body. The medical approach focuses on the biological organism and pathological processes. This model of disease has shown tremendous success when dealing for example with acute infectious diseases but has been less successful with chronic degenerative diseases such as heart disease and cancer. These diseases have many etiological causes and there is no known cure; they present a major challenge to the medical profession, one that has become heightened as the population ages because, as noted earlier, in old age we tend to suffer more from chronic conditions than we do from acute illnesses.

It is now more than half a century since the World Health Organization recognized the multifaceted nature of good health as "a state of complete physical, mental and social well-being and not merely the absence of disease or infirmity" (World Health Organization 1948:100). That is, it is more or less accepted today that health is multidimensional, including three interrelated dimensions: physical (the presence or absence of signs of disease and symptoms of illness); the psychological (feelings of well-being); and the social (the capacity to perform usual well roles typically measured in terms of one's functional ability with basic and instrumental activities of daily living).

All industrialized countries embraced a vision of health reform in the early 1990s that called for a broadening of health beyond a biomedical definition and that embraced the value of community care. Mahtre and Deber (1992) reviewed available reports from provincial and federal working groups established to examine the health care systems in Canada. They reported remarkable similarities among the reports which included:

- Broadening the definition of health to include aspects in addition to the biomedical, such as the social and psychological aspects with the collaboration of multiple sectors.
- Shifting the emphasis from curing illness to promoting health and preventing disease.
- Switching the focus to community-based care rather than institutional-based care.
- Providing more opportunities for individuals to participate with service providers in making decisions on healthy choices and policies.
- Decentralization of the provincial systems to some form of regional authorities.
- Improved human resources planning with particular emphasis on alternative methods for remuneration of physicians, other than fee-for-service.
- Enhanced efficiency in the management of services for the establishment of councils, coordinating bodies, and secretariats.
- Increasing the funds for health services research, especially in the areas of utilization.
- Technology assessment, program or system evaluation, and information systems.

That is, there was tremendous consistency in the vision of health reform to broaden the definition of health from a narrow biomedical perspective, to shift the focus from curative treatment to promoting health and preventing disease, and to changing the focus from institutional-based care to community-based care.

While it is argued elsewhere (Chappell et al., 2003) that health reform can be seen as regressing and not implementing this vision, that is not the task of this report. Rather, I would like to use the vision of health reform to talk about incorporating a health promotion perspective within health care systems throughout the world and about the implications for practice with seniors, if indeed we incorporated this direction. If we examine what health promotion is, it should become clear that this perspective is important when dealing with the mental health of seniors.

A HEALTH PROMOTION PERSPECTIVE

Health promotion begins by recognizing "upstream" factors as influencing our health. That is, it recognizes the role of psychosocial and environmental factors in health. This follows from a broad definition of health as "… a state of complete physical, mental and social well-being and not merely the absence of disease or infirmity" (World Health Organization, 1948). The Ottawa charter, emerging from the first international conference on health promotion, proclaims that health is the "process of enabling people to increase control over, and to improve, their health.". . . and "to reach a state of complete physical, mental and social well-being, an individual or group must be able to identify and realize aspiration, to satisfy needs, and to change or cope with the environment." Health determinants that are prerequisites for achieving health include: peace, shelter, education, food, income, a stable ecosystem, sustainable resources, social justice, and equity. Levin (1987) argues that lifestyle is the same as health promotion, consisting of a selective pattern of health promoting behaviors based on choices available to persons according to their life chances.

Indeed, research suggests that many Canadian seniors already engage in a health promotion perspective. For example, we know that seniors often engage in self-treatments simultaneously while under professional care (Segall & Chappell, 1991). Subcultural groups such as Chinese Canadian seniors often use both traditional and western medicine simultaneously (Chappell & Lai, 1998). Furthermore, seniors often normalize symptoms (vision problems, constipation, indigestion, sleeplessness) as simply part of normal aging (Stoller, 1993). Seniors though tend to not attribute chronic illness to aging but rather to biological or lifestyle factors (Blaxter, 1983). In addition, seniors who are ill and disabled can and often do consider themselves well. That is, one can be healthy in certain aspects but unhealthy in others.

Especially important in this perspective is the notion of a host response or the general susceptibility hypothesis (Evans & Stoddart, 1990). Contrary to a biomedical perspective, in which specific pathogenic causes are sought for different physiological conditions, the host response argues that the body can be generally susceptible to disease. That is, if we find a cure for cancer tomorrow, that individual will develop another illness. The implications of this notion are profound—for how we treat illness, for how we respond to illness, for how we approach prevention. This notion suggests we must take a holistic approach to prevention and care.

Taking a broad perspective, it is clear that there is room for improvement among Canada's elderly population. For example, the majority are sedentary—over 65% of those age 65 and over (Eakin, 2001), and this increases with age, to 70% of those who are age 75 and over. Seniors give a variety of reasons for this: medical condition, perception that the condition is a barrier, no interest, no motivation, no time, no companion or social support, no program (Satariano, Haight, & Tager, 2000), despite the fact that research demonstrates that physical activity can be beneficial even for those with severe medical conditions and who are chair bound. And the benefits accrue even when activity is begun late in life (Spirduso, 1995; Hickey & Stilwell, 1992). Diabetes is an illness example. The known risk factors for diabetes, as for other chronic illnesses, include obesity, poor nutrition, physical inactivity, and low socioeconomic status. Lifestyle modifications have been shown to work (Little, 2003; Whitaker, 2000).

The challenge, of course, is to translate this health promotion perspective into our models of health care and into practice within our health care systems and beyond. There is no shortage of proponents of a health promotion approach (Stokols, 1995; Stokols, Allen, & Bellinham, 1996; Merzel & D'Afflitti, 2003; Glasgow, Lichtenstein, & Marcus, 2003). And others have developed a Chronic Care Model (Wagner et al., 1999) across conditions as effective management strategies and demands placed on the health care system are similar irrespective of the cause of the particular chronic condition. Within the Chronic Care Model, patients are viewed as active participants in their own care, requiring broader support than solely biomedical interventions. Quality of life for patient and family are considered important outcomes.

In 2001, the World Health Organization published a modification of this model, the Innovative Care for Chronic Conditions (ICCC) Framework, recognizing the relevance of a broad policy environment. Guiding foci of this revision include: evidence based decision making; a population rather than individual focus; a quality focus; integration of various levels of the system; flexibility/adaptability; and a prevention focus because most chronic conditions are preventable. A further modification has created the Expanded Chronic Care Model (ECCM) to explicitly combine population health promotion and improved treatment of chronic disease (Barr et al., 2002). The ECCM recognizes the role of social determinants of health and the central role of community in creating healthy communities and advocates a porous border between the formal health care system and the community. The health care sector is seen as an essential partner in creating the proper conditions for health, in a leadership role by providing examples of what can be done and advocating for healthy public policies. For improved outcomes for chronic disease management, the health care system requires redesign, not simply additional interventions to the current system which is designed mainly to provide acute care.

That is, it is increasingly recognized that chronic disease care calls for a reorganization of the current health care system. Treatment and prevention call for action outside as well as inside the health care system. Often viewed as synonymous with health promotion, a population health approach focuses attention outside of the formal health care system to the entire range of individual and collective factors determining health (Hamilton & Bhatti, 1996; Health Canada, 2001). It focuses on the entire population not just a segment and not just those who are sick or at risk of being sick. It includes those who feel healthy as well as those who feel ill; it includes both personal and structural factors (social and economic factors such as living and working conditions) that determine health, not only traditional risk factors (biology, genetic endowment, and access to health services) related to diseases. The social determinants of health include personal health beliefs and self-care practices, social status in our various social situations, and supportive relationships. The structural elements in particular—work hierarchies, educational systems, family structure, recreational systems—are all difficult to change but draw attention to broader societal forces that impinge on our health, including our mental health. Such an approach forces attention on not only individuals and the formal health care system but also on larger units of analysis, groups, communities, whole societies and how they are organized.

We know that a health promotion and population health approach takes time and citizen involvement (Frank & Di Ruggiero, 2003). Nevertheless, interactions within the health care system also require preventive support. Indeed, the World Health Organization (2001) argues that this should be the case for every health care interaction. There is much that health care workers can do, both inside and outside of the health care system within which they work, and social workers, with a largely psychosocial perspective, have much to contribute through their practice.

IMPLICATIONS FOR PRACTICE

Recognizing that societal and system change takes time and that individuals working within the system can feel helpless in affecting that process, there are nevertheless actions that can be taken. Social workers in particular have a key role to play in the health promotion of seniors. Adapting a broadened view of health and taking into account more than the "illness reality" of seniors and their associated problems is paramount (Pullen, Noble Walker, & Fiandt, 2001). An overemphasis on the illness can result in a lack of attention to health practices that maintain wellness and prevent functional decline, resulting, especially among women, in their redefining their health and life negatively, with resulting defeatism and diminished capacity to cope (Lapp, 2000).

In order to focus on the social determinants of health, social workers need to build a social relationship and a sense of wholeness with the senior client (Gladden, 2000). This relates to the fact that telling people what to do is not enough. Information and education are important but insufficient to convince people of any age to change their lifestyles; this is also true of seniors. Support from family, friends, and age peers is important but support from health professionals is also important (Frohlich & Potvin, 1999; Haber et al., 2000). Simultaneously, there is a need for an equitable balance of knowledge, respect and power in the care relationship (McWilliam, Diehl-Jones, Jutai, & Tadrissi, 2000); a need to listen to what the client perceives as her/his needs. That is, health care professionals are not the only one with expertise.

Clients have expertise as well. This is particularly true when dealing with subcultural and ethnic beliefs and traditions of older clients. This speaks to empowerment of clients to take control over their own lives where feasible. Relatedly, social workers can assist clients by bringing together support groups for those with similar conditions and circumstances and for family members of clients. It is important though, that professionals not insert themselves into the process as the "expert" and treat participants as the "recipients" of this expert knowledge. If professionals are involved in the groups they must skillfully participate as facilitators.

Interventions designed to provide individuals with coping skills can lead to improved self-esteem and self-efficacy. Such strategies aim at building life skills that are generalizable to several areas of life and provide the foundation for enhancing overall quality of life.

Other than at the individual client interface, there are other opportunities for social workers to implement a health promotion perspective. Those in decision-making positions can explicitly work towards bringing in a health promotion perspective. An example would be the adoption of the recently developed Seniors Mental Health Policy Lens (McCourt, 2004), designed to develop the capacity of communities to use psychosocial approaches to promote seniors' mental health, to prevent and/or to address mental health problems. It was designed after wide consultation with practitioners, policy makers, researchers and seniors. It is designed for use by policy makers, program managers, designers, evaluators, clinicians, and seniors' advocacy groups. The policy lens questions are:

- Has the policy been developed in collaboration with those who will be most affected?
- Does the policy address the diverse needs, circumstances, and aspirations of vulnerable subgroups within the seniors' population? Are any negative effects from this policy likely to be magnified for any of these groups?
- Does the policy acknowledge the multiple determinants of health?
- Does the policy consider accessibility?
- Does the policy support seniors' social participation and relationships?
- Does the policy support seniors' independence and self-determination?
- Does the policy support seniors' dignity?
- Is the policy fair? Does it take into account the full costs and benefits of supporting the aspirations of seniors?
- Does the policy/program support seniors' sense of security?
- Is consideration given to the cumulative impacts on later life of policies/programs targeted at earlier life stages?

If taken seriously, such a simple, easy-to-use guide can assist policy and program designers.

In addition, the education of social workers could be revised, to ensure they are well versed in the social determinants of health. Continuing education is required to know the latest research in an area. Social workers also need to make explicit and be aware of their own personal biases that they may bring to their interactions with clients. The now familiar rhetoric about client-centeredness, consumers and empowerment is not necessarily translated into action. Indeed, some argue such words are motivated by a desire to transfer the responsibility and cost of care to consumers and their families (Walker, 1991), rather than by a genuine interest in the welfare of their clients.

CONCLUSIONS

This article has examined some of the health facts regarding aging, noting the physical decline in health as we age. However, psychological well-being, whether referring to aspects of physical health such as one's perceptions of physical health or to more psychological concepts such as life satisfaction and sense of coherence do not necessarily decline as we age. The discrepancy between the two highlights the importance of a broad holistic definition of health such as the one put forward by the World Health Organization over half a century ago. While the vision of health reform that emerged throughout the industrialized world in the 1990s is consistent with such a broadened view of health and allows one to take into account the discordance just noted, health care systems remain largely focused on a narrow biomedical approach to physical illness. Yet, the vision of health reform calls for heightened attention to a health promotion perspective. The upstream nature of health promotion with its recognition of the social determinants of health and of a population health perspective call for the inclusion of health as well as illness in a holistic treatment of individuals. Twenty-five years ago Antonovsky (1979) distinguished between pathogenesis (referring to the origins of disease) and salutogenesis (referring to the factors that protect and enhance good health). This distinction still requires attention. A health promotion perspective directs us to incorporate both into our thinking.

It would appear clear that a health promotion perspective has benefits for seniors with illnesses and disabilities as well as those who by and large are healthy. It has the potential to prevent decline as well as to ensure a less expensive health care system. A health promotion perspective however, requires a culture shift within the health care system and among health care professionals, especially those who are medically trained such as physicians and nurses. Social workers have a key leadership role to play in this shift given their greater psychosocial perspective than many other health care professionals. Furthermore, even though system change takes time and individual health care workers often feel and indeed are disempowered, individuals can make a difference both at the client interface and program and policy levels within and outside of the health care system.

REFERENCES

Antonovsky, A. (1979). *Health, Stress, and Coping*. San Francisco: Jossey-Bass Publishers.
Barr, V., Robinson, S., Marin-Link, B., Underhill, L., Dotts, A., & Ravensdale, D. (2002). The Expanded Chronic Care Model Summary. *Hospital Quarterly, 7*, (1).
Blaxter, M. (1983). The causes of disease: Women talking. *Social Science and Medicine, 17*, 59–69.

Canadian Study of Health and Aging (1994). The Canadian study of health and aging: Study methods and prevalence of dementia. *Canadian Medical Association Journal* *150*(6), 899–913.

Chappell, N.L., Gee, E., MacDonald, L., & Stones, M. (2003). *Aging in Contemporary Canada*. Toronto: Prentice Hall.

Chappell, N.L., & Lai, D. (1998). Health care service use among Chinese seniors in British Columbia, Canada. *Journal of Cross-Cultural Studies, 13*, 21–37.

Craik, F.I.M., & Jennings, J.M. (1992). Human memory. In F.I.M. Craik & T.A. Salthouse, (Eds.). *Handbook of aging and cognition* (pp. 51–110). Hillsdale, NJ: Erlbaum.

Eakin, E. (2001). Promoting physical activity among middle-aged and older adults in health care settings. *Journal of Aging and Physical Activity, 9*(Suppl.), S29–S37.

Elston, M.A. (1993). Women doctors in a changing profession: The case of Britain. In E. Riska & K. Wegar, (Eds.), *Gender, work and medicine: Women and the medical division of labour*, pp. 27–61. Newbury Park, CA: Sage Publications.

Evans, R.G., & Stoddart, G.L. (1990). Producing health, consuming health care. *Social Science & Medicine, 31*, 1347–1363.

Federal Provincial and Territorial Provincial Advisory Committee on Population Health, (1999). Ottawa, ON: Statistics Canada.

Frank, John, & Di Ruggiero, Erica (2003). Prevention: Delivering the Goods. *Longwoods Review, 1*(2).

Freidson, E. (1970). *Profession of medicine: A study of the sociology of applied knowledge*. New York: Dodd, Mead.

Frohlich, K.L., & Potvin, (1999). Collective lifestyles as the target for health promotion. *Canadian Journal of Public Health, 90* (Suppl. I), 1–14.

Gallo, J., Rabins, P., & Hopkins, J. (1999). Depression without sadness: Alternative presentations of depression in late life. *American Family Physician, 60*, 820–826.

Gladden, J.C., (2000). Information exchange: critical connections to older adult decision-making during health care transitions. *Geriatric Nursing, 21*(9), 9–15.

Glasgow, R.E., Lichtenstein, E., & Marcus, A.C. (2003). Why Don't We See More Translation of Health Promotion Research to Practice? Rethinking the Efficacy-to-Effectiveness Transition. *American Journal of Public Health, 93*(8), 1261–1267.

Gritzer, G. (1981). Occupational specialization in medicine: Knowledge and market explanations. *Research in the Sociology of Health Care, 2*, 251–283.

Hamilton, N., & Bhatti, T. (1996) *Population Health Promotion: An Integrated Model of Population Health and Health Promotion*. Ottawa, Canada: Health Canada.

Haber, D., Looney, C., Bobola, K., Hinman, M., & Utsey, C.J. (2000). Impact of a health promotion course on inactive, overweight, or physically limited older adults. *Family and Community Health, 22*(4), 48–56.

Health Canada. (2001) *The Population Health Template: Key Elements and Actions that Define a Population Health Approach*. Ottawa: Health Canada.

Hickey, T., & Stilwell, D.L. (1992). Chronic illness and aging: a personal contextual model of age-related changes in health status. *Educational Gerontology, 18*, 1–15.

Hultsch, D.F., Hertzog, C., Small, B.J., McDonald-Miszlak, L., & Dixon, R.A. (1992). Short-term longitudinal change in cognitive performance in later life. *Psychology and Aging, 7*, 571–584.

Lapp, C. (2000). What health means to older adults. *What's News*. Available at: http://www.ccp.uwoshe.edu/whatsnews/fall2000/healthview.html.

Levin, L.S. (1987). Every silver lining has a cloud: the limits of health promotion. *Social Policy, 27*, 57–60.

Little, D. (2003). Non-pharmacological management of diabetes: the role of diet and exercise. *Geriatrics & Aging, 6*(1), 27–29.

Mahtre, S.L., & Deber, R.B. (1992). From equal access to health care to equitable access to health: A review of Canadian provincial health commissions and reports. *International Journal of Health Services, 22*(4), 645–668.

McCourt, (2004). *Seniors mental health policy lens. www.seniorsmentalhealth.ca*, (report).

McWilliam, C.L., Diehl-Jones, W.L., Jutai, J., & Tadrissi, S. (2000). Care delivery approaches and seniors' independence. *Canadian Journal on Aging, 19*(Suppl. I): 101–124.

Merzel, C. & D'Afflitti, J. (2003). Reconsidering Community-Based Health Promotion: Promise, Performance, and Potential. *American Journal of Public Health, 93*(4), 557–574, April.

Myers, D.G., & Diener, (1995). Who is happy? *Psychological Science, 6*, 10–19.

Pullen, C., Noble Walker, S.N., & Fiandt, K. (2001). Determinants of health promoting lifestyle behaviors in rural older women. *Family and Community Health, 24*, (2), 49–72.

Reisberg, B., Ferris, S.H., deLeon, & Crook (1982). Relationships in late midlife *The Journal of Gerontology: Series B: Psychological Sciences and Social Sciences, 52B*(4), S170–S179.

Riska, E., & Weger, K. (1993). Women physicians: A new force in medicine? In E. Riska & K Wegar (Eds.), *Gender, work and medicine. Women and the medical division of labour (pp.27–61)*. Newbury Park, CA: Sage Publications.

Satariano, W.A., Haight, T.J. & Tager, I.B. (2000). Reasons given by older people for limitation or avoidance of leisure time physical activity. *Journal of the American Geriatrics Society, 48*(5), 505–512.

Segall, A., & Chappell, N.L. (2000). *Health and Health Care in Canada*. Toronto: Prentice Hall.

Segall, A., & Chappell, N.L. (1991). Making sense out of sickness: Lay explanations of chronic illness among older adults. *Advances in Medical Sociology, 2*, 115–133.

Schaie, K.W. (1996). *Intellectual Development in Adulthood: The Seattle Longitudinal Study*. New York: Cambridge University Press.

Spirduso, W.W. (1995). *Physical dimensions of aging*. Champaign, IL: Human Kinetics.

Statistics Canada: *www.hc-sc.gc.ca/seniors*, 2001.

Statistics Canada, Canadian Community Health Survey, Mental Health and Well-being - Cycle 1.2, 2002. Ottawa: Statistics Canada.

Statistics Canada, Canadian Community Health Survey (CCHS), 2000/01. Ottawa: Statistics Canada.

Statistics Canada, (1999). *A portrait of seniors in Canada*, (3rd Ed.). Ottawa: Statistics Canada Housing, Family and Social Statistics Division.

Stokols, D. (1995). Translating Social Ecological Theory into Guidelines for Community Health Promotion. *American Journal of Health Promotion 10*(4): 282–298.

Stokols, D., Allen, J., & Bellingham, R.L. (1996). The Social Ecology of Health Promotion: Implications for Research and Practice. *American Journal of Health Promotion 10*(4): 247–251.

Stoller, E. (1993). Interpretations of symptoms by older people. *Journal of Aging Health, 5*, 58–81.

Stones, M.J., & Kozma, A. (1980). Issues relating to the usage and conceptualization of mental health constructs employed by gerontologists. *International Journal of Aging and Human Development, 11*, 269–281.

Wagner, E.H., Davis, C., Schaefer, J., Von Korff, M. & Austin, B. (1999). Building a Health Care System for Chronic Conditions: The Innovative Care for Chronic Conditions Framework. *Managed Care Quarterly, 7*(3), 56–66.

Walker, A. (1991). The Relationship between the Family and the State in the care of Older People. *Canadian Journal on Aging. 10* (2), 94–112.

Whitaker, J. (2000). *Reversing hypertension*. New York, NY: Warner Brooks.

World Health Organization. (2001). Health aging adults with intellectual disabilities: summative report. *Journal of Applied Research in Intellectual Disabilities, 14*(3), 256–275.

World Health Organization. (1948). *Official records of the World Health Organization*, Number 2: WHO Interim Commission, United Nations. p.100.

Representations of Elderly with Mental Health Problems Held By Psychosocial Practitioners from Community and Institutional Settings

Bernadette Dallaire, PhD
Michael McCubbin, PhD
Normand Carpentier, PhD
Michèle Clément, PhD

THE SITUATION OF ELDERLY PEOPLE SUFFERING FROM MENTAL HEALTH PROBLEMS: PREVALENCE, CONSEQUENCES, AND SERVICES

Even if the elderly today are generally healthier than in the past, the mental health problems that they face are still important and growing due to the aging of the populations of Western societies.

Depression is estimated to affect 3% of community dwelling elderly, and almost 40% of those living in institutions (National Advisory Council on Aging, 1999). Assuming continued increases in life expectancy, projections for the first quarter of the 21st century show a dramatic increase in the number of cases of depression and dementia among elderly, since the risks of suffering from one of these problems increase with aging (LeClair & Sadavoy, 1998). Among North Americans 65 and older, 2% have been estimated to be suffering from severe mental illness [SMI] (severe anxiety disorders, chronic depression, schizophrenia and personality disorders) (Bartels, Levine, & Shea, 1999). Given the aging of the population, it is expected that the number of elderly with SMI will double in the next 30 years in North America (Bartels et al., 1999). Projections concerning schizophrenia are especially worrying: schizophrenia cases among the 55 + age group are projected to double by 2030 (Cohen et al., 2000).

Elderly people with mental health problems represent a population that is especially vulnerable. The addition of mental health problems with those associated with the process of aging has major consequences at the health, functional and psychosocial levels. This is especially true regarding seniors with SMI, for whom already severe vulnerability due to aging is further aggravated (Bartels et al., 1999; Bernstein & Hensley, 1993; Florio & Raschko, 1998). The presence of chronic or acute physical conditions related to old age aggravates vulnerability and can lead to further functional impairments, exacerbating existing mental health problems. With respect to elderly with SMI, the functional impairments can affect many important dimensions of their lives. Many elderly with SMI are socially isolated (Florio & Raschko, 1998), their social abilities are inadequate (Bartels et al., 2004) and, partly because of cognitive or physical comorbidity, their capacities for adaptation and problem solving are limited (Cohen, 2001). With respect to both seniors suffering from less severe or transitional psychological distress (e.g., situational depression) and seniors with SMI, the combination of aging and mental health problems can also lead to physical somatization, neglect of health needs (Bartels et al., 2004), suicidal ideations or acts, and to institutionalizations that are premature or otherwise preventable (Fogel, Furino, & Gottleib, 1990; Osgood, 1992). These problems and related consequences can severely jeopardize their capacity to continue to live in the community (Bartels et al., 2004).

Despite the importance of the needs of this population, several problems persist in the mental health services offered to them. Much research points to problems of underutilization and of access to services: generally, elders are reluctant to consult, or they do not consult because of limitations in their mobility (National Advisory Council on Aging, 1999; Waxman, 1986). With regards to older adults with SMI, the low rate of mental health services use has been related by some to a "lack of perceived need" (see Klap, Unroe, & Unutzer, 2003). However, a growing number of clinical and evaluation studies have stressed that even when seniors consult professionals (especially general practitioners and psychiatrists), there are considerable flaws in the identification of, and in the response to, mental health problems, notably: (1) nondiagnosis [e.g., symptoms of depression are undetected, or attributed by clinicians to the "normal profile" of old age], or erroneous diagnosis [e.g., simple insomnia instead of anxiety] (Mackenzie, Gekoski, & Knox, 1999; Waxman, 1986); and (2) prescription of psychotropic medication as the solution to situational problems [e.g., bereavement after the death of a spouse] (Krauss, 2005; Voyer, McCubbin, Préville, & Boyer, 2003), or inappropriate prescription or overprescription of psychotropics, especially in institutional settings such as nursing homes (Bronskill et al., 2004).

For some clinical analysts, the problems in the development of diagnostic ability and in the clinical response are directly related to a generally pessimistic attitude regarding the prognosis for elderly with mental health problems, which is often seen as "hopeless" by health care practitioners (Goldlist, 2000). Such a pessimism, and sense of inadequacy for effective provision of help, is also pervasive among other types of service providers, such as social workers (Kindiak, Grieve, Randall, & Madsen, 2004). In his seminal article about psychiatry and the elderly, Butler (1975) characterized this phenomenon as "therapeutic nihilism."

Globally, services are far from meeting the special needs of this population (Bartels, 2003). General long-term geriatric services are centered on clients suffering from physical impairments and cognitive deficits, and dedicate few resources to severe mental illnesses (Cohen, 2001). Existing psychological or gerontopsychiatric services often lack integration and put emphasis on pharmacological treatment and on acute or transitory conditions (Bartels et al., 1999, 2004; Cohen, 2001; Holmes, Bentley, & Cameron, 2003).

Furthermore, with regard to institutional settings, recent studies have shown both a tendency to overprescription of neuroleptic medication (Bronskill et al., 2004) and to under-referral for psychological or psychiatric consultation (Fenton et al., 2004). In fact, these studies reveal that both prescription of neuroleptics and psychological/psychiatric evaluation are related to behavioural problems/disturbances: it appears that "quiet" signs of distress (social withdrawal, lethargy) do not trigger a referral for mental health intervention, while "disturbing" behaviours make residents more prone to be medicated and/or referred for psychological or psychiatric intervention.

It appears that community services also are in need of improvement and/or better adaptation. In many jurisdictions, it is currently hard to "locate" the elderly clientèle in the organization of services. For instance, our consultations with fieldworkers in Quebec City and elsewhere in the province of Quebec, Canada, have indicated that elders with mental health problems and SMI are identified either as users of general geriatric services, or as users of general mental health services, and thus are merged with one of these two clientèles (Dallaire, McCubbin, Carpentier, & Clément, 2004). Consequently, a growing number of analysts are stressing the urgent need for models of community-based rehabilitation services specifically designed for elderly persons with SMI (Bartels et al., 2004).

PSYCHOSOCIAL APPROACHES IN MENTAL HEALTH INTERVENTION WITH THE ELDERLY: RECOVERY, EMPOWERMENT, AND SOCIAL INCLUSION

Theoretically, community mental health services designed for the elderly share some core orientations: (1) support provided in their natural living environments; (2) development and preservation of their autonomy; (3) taking into account the entire person and that person's environment, including medical, functional and psychosocial needs; and (4) integration into the community (Dallaire, Miranda, Moscovitz, & Guérette, 2003; Quebec Mental Health Committee, 1997; Quebec Ministry of Family and Childhood, 2001). These orientations are part of a broader path of psychosocial rehabilitation, an approach that is seen as effective on the preventive and curative levels for elderly people with mental health problems (Cohen, 2001; McInnis, 1997; Weiss & Lazarus, 1993), including those with SMI (Bartels et al., 2004). However, this kind of approach is too scarcely used in conventional mental health services delivered to elderly persons (Chiu, Yastrubetskaya, & Williams, 1999; D'Altilia, Moscovitz, Guérette, & Miranda, 2002).

The principles underlying the interrelated concepts of recovery, empowerment and social inclusion are at the heart of psychosocial intervention, both in mental health and in gerontology. We believe that their application is essential for optimizing the quality of life of elders suffering from transitional conditions and those with SMI, and for allowing them optimal management of their everyday life (Bartels, 2003; Chiu et al., 1999; Dallaire et al., 2004).

Recovery

Recovery, in the domain of mental health, is seen as a process in which a person tries to transcend a situation characterized by one or more of physical or mental impairments, functional limitations, or social handicap. The aim is that the person will be able to renew the meaning of his/her life and that this person will be able to perform her/his social roles (for two thorough reviews of the recovery literature, see Allott, Loganathan, & Fulford, 2002[2004]; and Provencher, 2002). Thus, recovery is not, by usual standards, a clinical/treatment-oriented concept. Because it reflects the point of view of the recovering individual instead of the clinician's, it constitutes a major departure from traditional biomedical notions such as "cure" or "symptoms." Recovery is a life course experience (thus not a "state" nor a "result") by which an individual's existence changes, both concretely and in its meaning. When used as an analytical tool, recovery is a central concept in the phenomenology of mental health, that is, the study of how the social world is subjectively experienced and thus interpreted by individuals (i.e., the "life-world"—see Moran, 2000, for a presentation of early general conceptualizations of the phenomenological approach; for a more contemporary application in mental health, see Scheff, 1999).

Empowerment

Empowerment is the process in which the individual develops his/her capacity to influence the organization and the course of his/her life. Such an influence is exercised mainly through decisions which directly affect the person, or which affect the community where he/she lives (Guttiérez, 1992; McCubbin & Cohen, 1996). In the empowerment process, decisions lead to actions, competencies and knowledge are developed and, in a dialectic with those processes, self-esteem increases (McCubbin, Cohen, & Dallaire, 2003).

Social Inclusion

Social inclusion provides the possiblity: (1) to be a member of social networks in which the individual performs meaningful roles and therefore experiences feelings of valorization and of belonging to a community; (2) to have the opportunity to access, and participate in, the basic functions of life in society (i.e., access to health care and to tools for recovery from incapacities, lodging, education, participation in meaningful activities which may include employment or volunteer work); and (3) to be involved as a citizen and a consumer (Billion, 1999; Castel, 1994). Here, we want to emphasize the importance of the resources coming from social networks, of the "regulation" that occurs during social interactions, and of daily interactions, the three having the potential to strengthen the bonds between the individuals, or alternatively, to impair or break these bonds in a process of exclusion (Carpentier & Ducharme, 2003).

Barriers to Implementation

Despite all the contemporary energy invested in the names of the principles of recovery, empowerment and social inclusion in current practice, important barriers still exist in mental health systems. Among these barriers, analysts identify:

(a) the limited role of clients in the design of mental health policies (Lord & Church, 1998; McCubbin & Cohen, 1996);

(b) the medicalization of problem definitions and of methods of intervention (Cohen, 1993; Kaufman, 1994), including in community services, which also remain dominated by medical model orientations (Baldwin, 1993; McCubbin et al., 2001);

(c) paternalistic approaches that augment and reinforce dependence and deresponsabilization among clients, who are seen as incompetent and vulnerable (Deegan, 1997; McCubbin et al., 2003; McCubbin & Cohen, 1999).

These barriers are all sociopolitical in nature, as observed by Carl Cohen (2001): "We must recognize that our views about outcome in the elderly with schizophrenia are determined as much by social and political factors as by clinical elements."

IMPACT OF SOCIAL REPRESENTATIONS IN PSYCHOSOCIAL INTERVENTION WITH ELDERLY CLIENTS WITH MENTAL HEALTH PROBLEMS

The preceding obstacles are sociopolitical and practical. They stem from a more fundamental obstacle, that is, a barrier pertaining to beliefs and perceptions: *disqualifying social representations* which aggravate the marginalization of the persons or impede their social inclusion. These disqualifying social representations concern both the elderly in general (Estes & Biney, 1991; Grant, 1996) and seniors who are affected by mental health problems (Dorvil & Benoit, 1999; Mendonça Lima et al., 2003; Waxman, 1986).

Social representation can be defined as a set of definitions, meanings, images, information, and attitudes regarding a given object (in the present case, elders with mental health problems, including SMI). Social representations orient the actions, social interactions, and communications carried out in a society. A representation is both a cognitive and a social phenomenon. A representation is social when: (1) it is shared by many members of a given society, community or group; (2) it is disseminated via communications involving members of a society/community/group (written messages, discourse, images); (3) its consequences are made visible through the actions that it inspires (visibility/observation of the enactment of a representation is, in this sense, a powerful form of dissemination of representations.); and (4) its construction and dissemination is strongly influenced by the social context—social norms, relations between groups, power inequalities, etc.—in which it emerges (see Abric, 1994; Dallaire, 1995[1997]; Herzlich, 1969; Huguet, 1996).

Because it helps to understand the relations between cognition and behavior at the individual and collective levels, the notion of social representation is a central analytical tool for understanding actions that take place in various settings, especially in professional practice. As we will discuss below, this is true with regards to interventions, programs, services, and policies regarding seniors with mental health problems.

Double Labelling ↔Double Stigmatization ↔Double Disqualification

Seniors suffering from mental health problems are subjected to a double labelling process in our societies: they are stigmatized both because of old age and because of mental illness (Bartels, 2003). This is especially the case for seniors suffering from SMI such as psychosis (Mendonça Lima et al., 2003). "Ageism"—i.e., negative stereotyping associated with old age (e.g., characterizing elderly persons primarily with assumptions of deterioration of physical and mental capacities, dependence, inability to adapt, general decline)—and the resulting discrimination against elders are now recognized as a pervasive phenomenon in current Western societies (Ragan & Bowen, 2002). With regards to mental illness, several empirical studies have documented the system of beliefs and practices which, in our cultures, organize the way we react to this condition: too often, interventions are based on a labelling of dangerousness to self or others (notably, that includes the notion of an inability to take proper care of oneself), and the belief in the necessity of control in addition to treatment (Angermeyer, Beck, & Matschinger, 2003; Clément, 2001), or of control to treat and treatment to control (Dallaire, McCubbin, Morin, & Cohen, 2000).

Literature regarding the general elderly population shows that organizations and professions are not immune to "ageism," which is said to be present in the policies, services and practices of health and social care institutions (Duerson, Thomas, Chang, & Stevens, 1992; Katz, 1990; Ward, 2000), with an obvious impact on how seniors' situations, needs, desires, goals and priorities are defined and responded to.

One can reasonably infer that this is especially true with regards to seniors suffering from mental illness, given the double stigma described above (Butler, 1975; Mendonça Lima et al., 2003; Waxman, 1986). However, there is a scarcity of scientific literature discussing the impact of the lay and professional representations regarding elderly persons suffering from mental health problems, that is, how these representations are actually enacted. But more fundamentally, there are no empirical studies of the very *nature* of these representations.

These considerations lead us to the following questions:

- What is the nature (contents, orientations, organization) of the representations elaborated by psychosocial practitioners working in institutional or community settings with regards to elderly people suffering from mental health problems?
- What is the relationship between lay and professional representations in these matters?
- What is the relationship between these representations and current psychosocial interventions?
- What is the relationship between these representations and the organizational contexts in which these psychosocial practices take place?
- What is the place of crucial notions such as recovery, empowerment and social inclusion in these representations?

We need to seek the answers to these questions to better understand professional practices, the systems of knowledge and beliefs supporting these practices, and the contexts in which practitioners evolve. By extension, the answers to these questions may contribute to better adapted psychosocial interventions in community and institutional settings. Especially, they would support the development and implementation of services, programs, and practices more oriented toward recovery, empowerment, and social inclusion. Such a change is required for better results in prevention and rehabilitation aimed at seniors suffering from mental health problems, a group that will expand dramatically, given the aging of the population in Western societies.

CONCLUSION

Our discussion demonstrates that despite calls for more adapted, more integrated, and more comprehensive services for elders suffering from mental health problems—especially calls for psychosocial interventions based on recovery, empowerment, and social inclusion approaches—several problems and barriers remain in the organization and delivery of services. In this chapter, we gave a special focus to obstacles pertaining to the way professionals define, interpret and assess the characteristics, situations, and needs of this segment of the population.

Literature about clinical practice reveals a misunderstanding of mental illness in older age and a pervasive pessimism in professional attitudes regarding seniors with mental illness. We can infer a relationship between these traits and the services-related problems mentioned above. By using the concept of social representations, we aim to go beyond this simple statement and to reach a deeper and more complete understanding of this relationship. Social representations are, by definition, both individual and collective phenomena. Their pervasiveness, persistence, and reproduction depend on their dissemination among citizens (including professionals), organizations, and institutions. They are also reinforced by their enactment, as performed by individuals, organizations, and institutions (on the institutional aspects, see Dallaire et al., 2000). We saw above that representations that convey stigma and social disqualification of elderly people with mental illness are, indeed, pervasive, persistent, and reproduced. We also saw that these representations are enacted—they have an impact on the way professionals respond to the needs of this segment of the population.

However, while the obvious focus of concern is how to intervene on the influence of representations on practices, we should not forget that the relationship between representations and actions is a two-way one: the way we act also determines the way we define/interpret/represent things or people. Moreover, our actions are also cumulative (we very rarely, if ever, act in a social vacuum), thus organized and institutionalized: to study—and to intervene on—representations of seniors suffering from mental illness is also, by extension, to tackle the organizational, institutional, and collective dimensions of the stigmatization and social exclusion that this particular group is subjected to.

REFERENCES

Abric, J.-C. (1994). Les représentations sociales: Aspects théoriques [social representations: theoretical aspects], In J.-C. Abric (Ed.), *Pratiques sociales et représentations* (pp. 11–36). Paris: PUF.

Allot, P., Loganathan, L., & Fulford, K.W.M. (2002[2004]). Discovering hope for recovery from a British perspective: A review of a selection of recovery literature, implications for practice and systems change. In S. Lurie, M. McCubbin, & B. Dallaire (Eds.), *Innovation in community mental health: international perspectives/Innovations en santé mentale communautaire: Perspectives internationales* [special issue]. *Canadian Journal of Community Mental Health/Revue canadienne de santémentale communautaire, 21*(3), 13–33.

Angermeyer, M.C., Beck, M., & Matschinger, H. (2003). Determinants of the public's preference for social distance from people with schizophrenia. *Canadian Journal of Psychiatry, 48*, 663–668.

Baldwin, S. (1993). *The myth of community care.* London: Chapman & Hall.

Bartels, S.J. (2003). Improving system of care for older adults with mental illness in the United States. Findings and recommendations for the President's New Freedom Commission on Mental Health. *American Journal of Geriatric Psychiatry, 11*, 486–497.

Bartels, S.J., Forester, B., Mueser, K.T., Miles, K.M., Dums, A.R., Pratt, S.I., Sengupta, A., Littlefield, C., O'Hurley, S., White, P., & Perkins, L. (2004). Enhanced skills training and health care management for older persons with severe mental illness. *Community Mental Health Journal, 40*, 75–90.

Bartels S.J., Levine K., & Shea, d. (1999). Community based long term care for older persons with severe and persistent mental illness in an era of managed care. *Psychiatric Services, 50*, 1189–1197.

Bernstein, M.A., & Hensley, R. (1993). Developing community-based program alternatives for the seriously and persistently mentally ill elderly. *Journal of Mental Health Administration, 20*, 201–207.

Billion, P. (1999). À propos de la notion d'intégration [on the notion of integration]. *Les Cahiers du Cériem, 4*, 3–24.

Bronskill, S.E., Anderson, G.M., Sykora, K., Wodchis, W.P., Gill, S., Shulman, K.I., & Rochon, P.A. (2004). Neuroleptic drug therapy in older adults newly admitted to nursing homes: Incidence, dose, and specialist contact. *Journal of the American Geriatrics Society, 52*, 749–755.

Butler, R.N. (1975). Psychiatry and the elderly: An overview. *American Journal of Psychiatry, 132*, 893–900.

Carpentier, N., & Ducharme, F. (2003). Caregiver network transformation: The need for an integrated perspective. *Ageing and Society, 23*, 507–525.

Castel, R. (1994). La dynamique des processus de marginalisation: De la vulnérabilité à la désaffiliation [dynamics of the marginalization process: from vulnerability to disaffiliation]. *Cahiers de recherche sociologique, 22*, 9–27.

Chiu, E., Yastrubetskaya, O., & Williams, M. (1999). Psychosocial rehabilitation of elderly with mental disorders: A neglected area in the psychiatry of old age. *Current Opinion in Psychiatry, 12*, 445–447.

Clément, M. (2001). L'exclusion des personnes atteintes de maladie mentale: Ancienne problématique, nouvelles réalités [the exclusion of people with mental illness: old problem definition, new realities] (pp. 489–509). In H. Dorvil & R. Mayer (Eds.), *Problémes sociaux, Tome 1: Théories et méthodologies.* Québec: Presses de l' Université du Québec.

Cohen, C.I. (1993). The biomedicalization of psychiatry: A critical overview. *Community Mental Health Journal, 29*, 509–521.

Cohen, C.I. (2001). Schizophrenia and the aging population. *Psychiatric Times, 18*(12). Available: http://www.psychiatrictimes.com/p011237.html

Cohen, C.I., Cohen, G.D., Blank, K., Gaitz, C., Katz, I.R., Leuchter, A., Maletta, G., Meyer, B., Sakauye, K., & Shamoian, C. (2000). Schizophrenia and older adults. An overview: Directions for research and policy. *American Journal of Geriatric Psychiatry, 8,* 19–28.

Dallaire B. (1995[1997]). Définir et reconnaître: Représentations de la santé et de la maladie dans trois départements hospitaliers [to define and to recognize: Representations of health and illness in three hospital wards]. *Health & Canadian Society/Santé et société canadienne,* 71–98.

Dallaire, B., McCubbin, M., Carpentier, N., & Clément, M. (2004). *Les représentations des problématiques gérontologie-santémentale chez les intervenants psychosociaux des milieux institutionnels et communautaires* [representations of problématiques gerontology-mental health among psychosocial practitioners from institutional and community settings]. Research funding submission to the Canadian Social Sciences and Humanities Research Council.

Dallaire B., McCubbin, M., Morin, P., & Cohen, D. (2000). Civil commitment due to mental illness and dangerousness: The union of law and psychiatry within a treatment-control system. *Sociology of Health and Illness, 22,* 679–699.

Dallaire B., Miranda, D., Moscovitz, N., & Guérette, A. (2003). *Les interventions communautaires auprés des personnes âgées aux prises avec des troubles mentaux graves: Revue critique de la littérature empirique et théorique* [community interventions with elders suffering from severe mental disorders: a critical review of empirical and theoretical literature]. Report submitted to the Quebec Foundation for Society and Culture. Québec: Bibliothéque nationale du Québec.

D'Altilia, L., Moscovitz, N., Guérette, A., & Miranda, D. (2002). La réhabilitation psychosociale des personnes âgées aux prises avec des problémes sévéres de santémentale. Au-delà du diagnostic [psychosocial rehabilitation of elders with severe mental health problems: beyond diagnosis]. Presentation to the XIème congrès de l' Association québécoise de réhabilitation psychosociale, Mont-Tremblant, Québec.

Deegan, P.E. (1997). Recovery and empowerment for people with psychiatric disabilities. *Social Work in Health Care, 25,* 11–24.

Dorvil H., & Benoit, M. (1999). Représentations sociales et conditions de vie despersonnes âgées classées malades mentales ou déficientes intellectuelles en résidence d'accueil [social representations and living conditions of elders labelled as mentally ill or mentally handicaped and living in nursing homes]. *Santé mentale au Québec, 14,* 228–252.

Duerson, M.C., Thomas, J.W., Chang, J., & Stevens, C.B. (1992). Medical students' knowledge and misconceptions about aging: Responses to Palmore's facts on aging quizzes. *Gerontologist, 32,* 171–174.

Estes C.L., & Biney, E.A. (1991). The biomedicalization of aging: Dangers and dilemmas. In M. Minkler & C.L. Estes (Eds.), *Critical perspectives of aging: The political moral economy of growing old* (pp. 117–134). New York: Baywood.

Fenton, J., Raskin, A., Gruber-Baldini, A., Srikumar Menon, A., Zimmerman, S., Kaup, B., Loreck, D., Ruskin, P.E., & Magaziner, J. (2004). Some predictors of psychiatric consultation in nursing home residents. *American Journal of Geriatric Psychiatry, 12*, 297–304.

Florio E.R., & Raschko, R. (1998). The Gatekeeper Model: Implications for social policy. *Journal of Ageing and Social Policy, 10*, 37–55.

Fogel, B.S., Furino, A., & Gottleib, G. (1990). *Mental health policy for older Americans: Protecting minds at risk.* Washington, DC: American Psychiatric Press.

Goldlist, B. (2000). Mental health management is no waste of clinical acumen: Prognosis for elderly patients is as favourable as for younger ones. *Geriatrics and Aging, 3*(4). Available: http://www.geriatricsandaging.ca/fmi/xsl/article.xsl?-lay = Article& Name = Mental%20Health%20Management%20is% 20No%20Waste% 20of %20Clinical %20 Acumen&-find

Grant, L.D. (1996). Effects of ageism on individual and health care providers' responses to healthy aging. *Health and Social Work, 21*, 9–15.

Guttiérez, L.M. (1992). Information and referral services: The promise of empowerment. *Information and Referral, 13*, 1–18.

Herzlich, C. (1969). Information and referral services: The promise of empowerment. *Information and Referral, 13*, 1–18.

Herzlich, C. (1969). *Santé et maladie: analyse d'une représentation social* [health and illness: Analysis of a social representation]. Paris: Mouton.

Holmes, J., Bentley, K., & Cameron, I. (2003). A UK survey of psychiatric services for older people in general hospitals. *International Journal of Geriatric Psychiatry, 18*, 716–721.

Huguet, P. (1996). Social representations as dynamic social impact. *Journal of Communication, 46*(4), 57–63.

Katz, S.R. (1990). Interdisciplinary geronotology education: Impact on multidimensional attitudes toward aging. *Gerontology and Geriatrics Education, 10*(3), 91–100.

Kaufman, S.R. (1994). Old age, disease, and the discourse on risk: Geriatric assessment in US health care. *Medical Anthropology Quarterly, 8*, 430–447.

Kindiak, D.H., Grieve, J.L., Randall, G.E., & Madsen, V.A. (2004). Social work practice in community psychogeriatric programs. In M.J. Holosko & M.D. Feit (Eds.), *Social Work with the Elderly. 3d Ed.* Toronto: Canadian Scholars' Press.

Klap, R., Unroe, K.T., & Utzer, J. (2003). Caring for mental illness in the United States: A focus on older adults. *American Journal of Geriatric Psychiatry, 11*, 517–524.

Krauss, R. (2005). Depression, antidepressants and an examination of epidemiological changes. *Radical Psychology Journal, 6*(1). Available: http://www.radpsynet.org/journal/

Leclair, J., & Sadavoy, J. (1998). Geriatric psychiatry subspecialization in Canada: Past, present and future. *Canadian Journal of Psychiatry, 43*, 681–687.

Lord J., & Church, K. (1998). Beyond "partnership shock": Getting to 'yes', living with 'no'. *Canadian Journal of Rehabilitation, 12*, 113–121.

Mackenzie, C.S., Gekoski, W.L., & Knox, V.J. (1999). Do family physicians treat older patients with mental health disorders differently from younger patients? *Canadian Family Physician, 45*, 1219–1224.

McCubbin M., & Cohen, D. (1996). Extremely unbalanced: Interest divergence and power disparities between clients and psychiatry. *International Journal of Law and Psychiatry, 19*, 1–25.

McCubbin M., & Cohen, D. (1999). A systemic and value-based approach to strategic reform of the mental health system. *Health Care Analysis, 7*, 57–77.

McCubbin M., Cohen D., & Dallaire, B. (2003). *Obstacles à l' empowerment en travail social: Vers un changement professionnel dans les interventions en santé mentale/* Empowering practice in mental health social work: Barriers and challenges. GRASP Working Papers Series, 30, 31. Montréal: Groupe de recherche sur les aspects sociaux de la santé et de la prévention. Available: http://www.grasp.umontreal.ca/documents/WP-Fr-30.pdf (français), http://www.grasp.umontreal.ca/documents/WP-An-31.pdf (English).

McCubbin, M., Weitz, D., Spindel, P., Cohen, D., Dallaire, B., & Morin, P. (2001). Submission for the President's Consultation regarding Community Mental Health Services. *Radical Psychology Journal, 2*(2). Available: http://www.radpsynet.org/journal/vol2-2/submission-mccubbin.html

McInnis, K. (1997). Empowerment-oriented mental health intervention with elderly Appalachian women: The Women's Club. *Journal of Women and Aging, 9*, 91–105.

Mendonça Lima, C.A., Levav, I., Jacobsson, L., Rutz, W., World Health Organization/ European Regional Office, Task Force on Destigmatization (2003). Stigma and discrimination against older people with mental disorders in Europe. *International Journal of Geriatric Psychiatry, 18*, 679–682.

Moran, D. (2000). *Introduction to phenomenology.* New York: Routledge.

National Advisory Council on Aging (1999). *1999 and after: Challenges for an aging society.* Ottawa: Government of Canada.

Osgood, N.J. (1992). *Suicide in later life: Recognizing the warning signs.* New York: Lexington.

Provencher, H.L. (2002). L'expérience du rétablissement: perspectives théoriques (the experience of recovery: theoretical perspectives). *Santé mentale au Québec, 1*, 35–64.

Quebec Mental Health Committee (1997). *Défis de la reconfiguration des services en santé mentale: Pour une réponse efficace et efficiente aux besoins des personnes atteintes des troubles mentaux graves et persistants* [challenges of reconfiguration of mental health services: for an effective and efficient response to the needs of people with severe and persistent mental disorders]. Québec: Ministère de la santé et des services sociaux.

Quebec Ministry of Family and Childhood (2001). *Le Québec et ses aînés: Engagés dans l'action. Engagements et perspectives 2001–2004* [Quebec and its seniors: commitments and prospects]. Québec: Gouvernement du Québec.

Ragan, A.M., & Bowen, A.M. (2002). Improving attitudes regarding the elderly population: The effects of information and reinforcement for change. *The Gerontologist, 41*, 511–515.

Scheff, T. (1999). *Being mentally ill: A sociological theory.* New York: de Gruyter.

Voyer P., McCubbin, M., Préville, M., & Boyer R. (2003). Factors in duration of anxiolytic, sedative and hypnotic use by elderly, and implications for nursing. *Canadian Journal of Nursing Research, 35*(4), 126–149.

Ward, D. (2000). Ageism and the abuse of older people in health and social care. *British Journal of Nursing, 9*, 560–593.

Waxman, H.M. (1986). Community mental health care for the elderly: A look at the obstacles. *Public Health Report, 101*, 294–300.

Weiss L.J., & Lazarus L.W. (1993). Psychosocial treatment of the geropsychiatric patient. *International Journal of Geriatric Psychiatry, 8*, 95–100.

Intensive Youth Outreach in Mental Health: An Integrated Framework for Understanding and Intervention

Victoria Ryall, BbSc, BSW, GradDip, MA
Sandra Radovini, MBBS, DPM, FRANZCP, Child Cert. RANZCP
Lee Crothers, B OT
Carsten Schley, DiplDipPsych
Karen Fletcher, BbSc, BSW
Simon Nudds, BSocSci, MSocSci, PGDipPsych
Cate Groufsky, BcNS

This article describes the major theories influencing the model of care for the Intensive Mobile Youth Outreach Service (IMYOS). ORYGEN Youth Health is mentioned as the service context for IMYOS, which is committed to the enhancement of clinical standards in the mental health care of young people. IMYOS has focused on the development and delivery of best practice interventions and has developed this model of care over seven years of clinical practice.

While this approach with young people does not as yet have a documented evidence base, this paper reviews the theoretical framework that informs clinical practice. A brief discussion of another Intensive Outreach Model with some empirical support is included as it also advocates the need for treatment to include family and other supports. This paper focuses on integrating four major theoretical paradigms. Each theory will be discussed briefly with respect to working with high-risk and difficult-to-engage young people. The inclusion of each has been influenced by the clinical presentation of the young people seen by IMYOS.

SERVICE CONTEXT

IMYOS arose out of a climate of growing community awareness about the needs of young people (aged between 12–24) in the Australian state of Victoria at significant risk of, in particular, homelessness, suicide, drug abuse, and unemployment. IMYOS offers Child and Adolescent Mental Health Services an enhanced community-based intensive model that targets those young people who had traditionally been difficult to engage in mainstream service delivery.

The IMYOS team provide an intensive, outreach mental health service to young people, their family, and the system. The young people seen by IMYOS are experiencing mental health difficulties and are unable to be adequately treated by a clinic-based program. Many of the young people seen by IMYOS have had extensive histories with multiple services such as (child) Protective Services and they are often not attending school or any other day program. They are likely to be experiencing family conflict and may live outside the family home. Many young people seen by IMYOS frequently present in crisis but appear to find proactive, regular help-seeking very difficult. Moreover, mental health difficulties and numerous psychosocial stressors usually compound these experiences.

IMYOS is a subprogram of ORYGEN Youth Health, a mental health service targeting early detection and treatment for young people aged 15–24 through clinical practice, research, and promotional activities.

IMYOS is a multidisciplinary team working intensively with complex clients. The team accept referrals from within the mental health system of Western Metropolitan Melbourne, Australia. Over a 12-month period, IMYOS received 38 referrals, 85% of which (19 female and 13 male) were accepted for treatment. The most prevalent diagnoses were Borderline Personality Disorder Traits, Major Depressive Disorder, Conduct Disorder, and Substance Abuse Disorders. Of the 32 accepted, 85% presented with more than one diagnosis.

IMYOS is staffed by two Psychologists, two Social Workers, one Occupational Therapist, and one Psychiatric Nurse. A Consultant Psychiatrist works two days a week. Each full-time clinician carries a caseload of 8–9 young people.

INTENSIVE PROGRAMS WITH YOUNG PEOPLE

There are few treatment approaches described in the literature for these complex young people. One approach described by Henggeler et al. (1998; 1999) outlines Multisystemic Therapy (MST) which incorporates intensive home- and community-based interventions that include the young person, their family, and local community. MST proposes that interventions with these complex young people require multifaceted interventions (Henggeler et al., 1999). Drawing on this work, the current model aims to provide a framework to guide necessarily flexible interventions for young people who are difficult to engage. IMYOS interventions are multifaceted and occur at three levels; individual, family, and systems (the other professionals/people involved in providing care to a young person).

FRAMEWORK

Figure 1 depicts the integration of theoretical concepts that have been influential in the development of the IMYOS treatment model. The first tier represents the overarching influence of developmental theory in IMYOS work. The second tier describes the theories that influence IMYOS conceptualisations of the difficulties young people present with. In accordance with Henggeler et al. (1999), this acknowledges the multidetermined nature of young people's difficulties. Each of these second tier theories highlights the importance of the therapeutic relationship. IMYOS considers the therapeutic relationship the fundamental tool of intervention. The third tier describes influential examples of how we may construct the therapeutic relationship.

The integration of these ideas is developed on a case-by-case basis and aids conceptualization of the young person and guides the treatment required. IMYOS works within a case management system, which can offer interventions varying from practical support to structured therapy. The team routinely employs treatment approaches such as Cognitive Therapy (Beck, 1995), Cognitive Analytic Therapy (Ryle & Kerr, 2002) or Narrative Therapy (White, 1999; White, 2000).

Literature exploring these areas is extensive and each paradigm has emerged from a variety of theories and philosophies. While thorough exploration of these perspectives is beyond the scope of this paper, aspects most relevant to IMYOS work will be briefly considered.

FIGURE 1. Theoretical Framework of IMYOS.

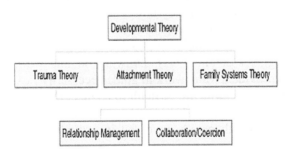

DEVELOPMENTAL THEORY

Consideration of the developmental trajectory of the young people seen by IMYOS is fundamental to our treatment approach. Developmental approaches make use of the chronological age of people to understand human behaviour. There are numerous theories that fall into this category including Freudian theory, Eriksonian theory, learning theory, and Piaget's theory, to name a few (Peterson, 1996). Each theory emphasizes different aspects of development and therefore differing practical applications. The common aspect of the theories is that people progress through various stages of development, each stage comprising different tasks and psychological needs. A central tenet of developmental theories is that marked deviations from the "norm" can highlight areas of difficulty (or strength) and can therefore assist in guiding back to a normative developmental trajectory (Steinhauer & Rae-Grant, 1983).

Developmental Theory and IMYOS

The influence of developmental theory within IMYOS is twofold. First, developmental characteristics of the young person must be considered. Adolescence and young adulthood are particularly significant periods of development because of the marked transitions in biological, psychological, and social systems during this time (Feldman & Elliot, 1990; Holmbeck & Updegrove, 1995). IMYOS considers that it is essential to be sensitive to developmental norms and levels, as well as the cognitive and emotional capabilities of clients, in order to deliver effective treatment. For example, we would expect that the cognitive and emotional ability of a 12-year-old to talk about a traumatic life event is likely to be very different from the capability of a 22-year-old, thus influencing the treatment approach. In general, IMYOS would choose a more behaviorally oriented treatment approach for younger clients and integrate more cognitive elements in work with older clients.

The onset of mental illness can derail the normal developmental trajectory of adolescence and young adulthood. Typical developmental appointments of young people, such as employment, education, and social and sexual relationships may have been interrupted or postponed. The task of the IMYOS clinician is to encourage re-engagement with these developmental tasks. For example, IMYOS case management often focuses on assisting a young person to reintegrate into school.

Second developmental theory influences IMYOS's understanding of the clients' presentation in the context of past (beneficial and adverse) experiences. Research has shown that critical incidents such as early separation from the primary carers or traumas (i.e., physical or sexual abuse) can have significant impact on the development of a young person and can influence the quality of future well-being and functioning (Lewis, 1996; Masten & Coatsworth, 1998; Cicchetti & Rogosch, 2002). Experiences will impact differently depending on the young person's level of development at the time these occurred. Furthermore, this impact will vary throughout the ongoing development. Adverse and beneficial experiences become part of a young person's developmental history and form a part of his/her resources and coping style. Thus, IMYOS considers the young person's developmental history alongside current influences and developmental challenges. The model also considers that the effects of early development are not immutable. Individual choice and subsequent experience (i.e., within therapy) can alter the course of development.

TRAUMA THEORY

This section will discuss and explore the dominance of traumatic experiences in the IMYOS population, the definition of trauma, the varying impact of trauma including its short and long term effects and the treatment implications for the individual, their family and system.

Dominance of Traumatic Experiences in the IMYOS Population

A significant majority of clients referred to IMYOS have histories of trauma and abuse, which is conceptualized as continuing to negatively affect their lives in a number of domains (i.e., individual, family, and system). While not all people who experience traumatic events suffer pathological and problematic outcomes, the experience of trauma alongside other factors appears to have a significant impact. Given the numerous psychosocial stressors experienced by many young people seen by IMYOS, the experience of trauma may have a profound impact.

Definition of Trauma

Traumatic events have been characterized by the DSM-IV (American Psychiatric Association, 1994) as involving the experience, witnessing, or confrontation of acutal or threatened death, serious injury, or threat to the physical integrity of self or others. Research has suggested that human-made traumatic events, with high levels of acute or chronic exposure to traumatic events in early development, trauma from a family member, concurrent difficulties, and histories of multiple victimization experiences are more likely to result in lasting psychological trauma and further pathological changes (Baum, 1987, cited in Davidson, Inslicht, & Baum, 2000; Fergusson, Lynskey, & Horwood, 1996; Guthrie & Notgrass, 1992). The most frequently occurring traumatic events/stressors reported by the IMYOS client population are typically of human-made origin and can be both acute and chronic. These include childhood sexual and/or physical abuse by a family member, neglect, being the recipient of or witnessing violence, sexual assault/rape as a young adult, and other multiple victimization experiences.

The Varying Impact of Trauma

Trauma is conceptualized as affecting an individual on a variety of levels, with complex interrelationships between psychological, biological, and social systems and processes (van der Kolk & McFarlane, 1996; Pynoos, Steinberg & Piacentini, 1999). The impact is mediated by variables such as the developmental level of the individual, the pretrauma vulnerability, the nature of the trauma (i.e., natural event vs. human origin), the length of time exposed to the traumatic event, and the family and community circumstances (Shalev, 1996; van der Kolk & McFarlane, 1996). Central to this framework is an awareness of the nature of traumatic memory and its neurobiological substrates (e.g., physiological hyperarousal) that lead to the dominance of the traumatic event(s) in memory and to its maintenance over time (van der Kolk, 1996). IMYOS clinicians consider the impact of trauma at each level and work with the factors that may moderate impact on current trauma processing.

Responses to traumatic events experienced by IMYOS clients may be mild and short-lived or chronic and pathological (and may be associated with acute stress reactions and PTSD symptomatology). Short-term effects of trauma are most commonly emotional or cognitive symptoms such as fear/anxiety, panic, emotional numbing, intrusive images of the traumatic event, and confusion or dissociation (Shalev, 1996). Young people present with initial effects such as behavioral problems, eating disturbances, and symptoms of hyperarousal such as problems sleeping (O'Donohue, Fanetti & Elliott, 1998).

Long-term effects of trauma include difficulties in regulating affect, aggression against self or others, problems with social attachments and intimacy, inability to trust others, social avoidance and isolation, and alterations in cognitive neurobiological processes (van der Kolk, 1996). These effects extend beyond strictly psychological and behavioral issues. The social sequelae of trauma (seen commonly in IMYOS clients) include isolation, increased interpersonal conflict, feelings of detachment and generally poor occupational and social functioning (Fergusson et al., 1996; O'Donohue et al., 1998; van der Kolk, 1996). In addition, the neurobiological impact of trauma can include biochemical and structural changes in the brain (Golier & Yehuda, 2002; Schwartz & Perry, 1994; van der Kolk, 1996). Trauma is remembered in the body and neuroana-tomical structures in the brain (van der Kolk, 1996). In addition, traumatic experiences have been shown to change subsequent cognitive and infor-mation processing systems (Golier & Yehuda, 2002; van der Kolk & McFarlane, 1996). Cognitive problems can include activation of threat-oriented cognitive schemas and distortions of thinking containing assumptions about the dangerous nature of the environment, other people and cognitive distortions such as minimizing safety-related events and maximizing threat-related, negative events.

Implications for Intervention

Central to the process of IMYOS treatment with the individual is the quality of the therapeutic relationship. Re-establishing a sense of personal safety is one of the primary goals of treatment with IMYOS clients. General therapeutic strategies such as collaboration, consistency, and validation can be useful to guide the client into a more adaptive therapeu-tic relationship. The development of safety plans are also important to establish the safety of the client (if self-harm or suicidal behavior is present).

Treatments such as anxiety management training and exposure therapies can be used to address the varied psychological and behavioral problems presented by the client. Cognitive therapy can assist the client to challenge their assumptions/thoughts relating to dangerousness, hyper-arousal, affective dysregulation, disassociation, and avoidance (Blake & Sonnenberg, 1998; Wagner & Linehan, 1998). IMYOS may also make use of a relational therapy in developing an understanding with a young person that helps them make sense of their current relational patterns (Ryle & Kerr, 2002). Psychoeducation for the young person, their family and other professionals is routine in IMYOS work. In relation to trauma this can include detailing aspects of biological impact and associated symptoms, which may aid family members (and others) to understand a young person's responses to trauma-related stimuli. IMYOS has under-taken family work focusing on the trauma of family members, which may be directly or indirectly related to that of the young person. Professionals may have their own reactions to the traumatic history of a young person (and/or its behavioural effects), which may impact on the clients move towards recovery. Therefore systems work may also involve facilitating professionals'[1] explorations of their own experience of working with the traumatized client and its impact on the working relationship. In summary, psychoeducation can assist all parties in developing an understanding and, importantly, a shared framework to understand the young person's situation.

ATTACHMENT THEORY

This section will outline briefly the main premise of attachment theory as it relates to IMYOS work and the dominance of this issue in young people seen by IMYOS. It will then explore the impact of problematic attachments for young people and IMYOS clients and, finally, discuss the implications for treatment in working with people who have experienced problematic attachments.

Attachment Theory and IMYOS

Attachment theory posits that early relationships with primary caregivers provides a template for relationships with others in life. John Bowlby, who formulated Attachment Theory, argued that "many forms of psychiatric disturbance can be attributed either to deviations in the development of attachment behaviour or, more rarely, to failure of its development" (Bowlby, 1979, p. 127).

A majority of the young people seen by IMYOS have had major disruptions in their early relationships with their primary caregiver, and many have received "pathological care" (neglect physical or sexual abuse by caregivers, removal or absence of caregiver, and/or having multiple caregivers).

Impact of Attachment Difficulties

When attachment is not secure or severely disrupted, the young person may repeatedly replicate insecure attachments with others. The DSM-IV describes lack of attachment that results in functional impairment, beginning prior to 5 years of age and associated with grossly pathological care (American Psychiatric Association, 1994) as reactive attachment disorder. These early experiences affect the lack of security in subsequent relationships. For example, a young person may repeatedly tell another to "leave them alone" which in turn results in the other giving up, thereby perpetuating their lack of a connected attachment. Attachment theory suggests that young people who are difficult to engage are not "bad" or "hopeless" but inexperienced in positive and trusting relationships and therefore avoidant of them. Attachment theory posits that the infant-parent relationship form the basis of mental life and relatedness and is the foundation of adult mental health (Lanyado, 2001). For example, if a child has little experience of reflective, reciprocal relationships that meet their emotional needs then this child will have very little sense of self and may persent with behavioural difficulties and/or mental health difficulties when older. Attachment insecurity or disturbances have been linkend to psychiatric syndromes, criminal behaviour and drug use (Shepheris, Renfro-Michel, & Doggett, 2003).

Implications for Intervention

Attachment theory offers the IMYOS model an understanding of young people's relational behavior and provides a base for formulating therapeutic interventions. IMYOS draws from attachment theory the understanding that a respectful, caring, and stable therapeutic relationship with someone can be reparative. It is suggested that the therapeutic relationship may provide an insight into the past experiences of care and current relationship building practices of the young person. For example, the clinician would hypothesize and may suggest to a young person who has had multiple losses of caregivers that it may be difficult to engage with someone for fear of experiencing another loss or seeing it as rejection.

IMYOS work is guided by an attachment framework to provide a safe relationship with young people that allows the young person to get feedback of how they appear in the relationship. This can aid the development of their sense of self, leading to improved mental health. IMYOS also puts strategies in place to foster relationships important to the young person, e.g., working towards a stable relationship between mother and daughter. The clinician may provide an outlet for the mother to express her anxieties, giving her more opportunity to be emotionally available to her daughter.

FAMILY/SYSTEMS THEORY

Many young people seen by IMYOS appear to have developed difficulties (and strengths) in the context of their family, and their behaviour may reflect family issues and dynamics (Dembo & Schmeider, 2002). Conceptualizations such as these have led to wider acceptance that effective interventions with young people must involve the family. This section will outline the family systems theory in relation to IMYOS. It will then elaborate on a family systems perspective on the family and individual functioning, and finally discuss the implications of this view for intervention.

Family Systems Theory and IMYOS

One of the basic notions accepted within the IMYOS model to understand family and individual interactions is that experience is relationally derived. Our first and often strongest relational experiences are within the family and begin before we are even aware of them (Dembo & Schmeidler, 2002). A family is usually a child's first "social" experience and it lays the foundations for all future "relational" acts. If relationships within a family system are problematic, the development and experience of relationships for an individual will be affected. Difficult relationship styles can develop and continue throughout the generations of the family, as this is where primary observation and learning occurs. A product of these problematic relationships, and the resulting poorly constructed coping mechanisms and communication styles, can perpetuate difficulties within the family (Ackerman, 1966). IMYOS clinicians assume that family members are doing the best they can in the circumstances. Additionally, the families seen by IMYOS have often experienced trauma and similar difficulties to the young person identified as the "client." It is essential to address the family system difficulties as well as treating the individual client. Clinicians need to understand a family's relational style and ways of interacting and communicating so that an individuals behaviours and difficulties can be understood and addressed in this context. It is critical to be mindful of the impact that family dynamics have on an individual and the need to address these family issues in order for individual change to occur.

Family Systems View of Individual and Family Difficulties

Minuchin's theory of family systems is employed within the IMYOS model to understand family functioning (Minuchin, 1974). In family groups all members influence and are influenced by every other member creating a system with unique properties. These properties are rules under which the family functions, and they aim to return the family to homeostasis

(Minuchin, 1974). Each family member has an interacting role to maintain this functioning. Symptoms or difficulties of one family member are viewed as relational rather than contained exclusively within the individual (Minuchin, 1974). This understanding can be used to explain to individuals that they are not solely to blame for the difficulties they experience. A family systems conceptualization suggests that the burden of change is shared, as problems can be seen to belong to the family system and not only the responsibility of the individual (Minuchin, 1974). This notion of shared responsibility can be difficult for some families to accept as the culture and burden of blame is very strong. The concept of "relationally derived difficulties" can be hard to understand and accept, particularly as parents fear being blamed for the difficulties their child presents with (and may in fact have experienced feeling blamed). Informing the family that each family member can play a key role in the change process may move a family away from blame.

Implications for Intervention

IMYOS often allocates a second team member to work with the family. It is helpful to separate the roles of individual and family worker so that clinicians are able to clearly define their roles with little confusion between individual and family issues. Each part of the "system" is recognized as having their own needs that should be addressed separately. Additionally, clinicians work to educate family members about the way that IMYOS seeks to construct a relationship with a young person, particularly in allowing them to make choices and, therefore, mistakes. The clinician will attempt to explain the importance of attachment figure. Clinicians have found that effective family oriented interventions can occur without a commitment from all family members. When an individual client will not engage with a worker we have found that engaging the family system may be the only avenue for intervention. Clear, supportive, and improved family relationships are of central importance in the reparatory experience for the individual.

IMYOS clinicians routinely attempt to actively involve family members in all aspects of treatment. This includes participation in the creation of a safety plan (a collaborative plan usually detailing how people will support a young person when they are unable to keep themselves safe) and consideration of how each family member can help intervene in an effective manner. A difficulty that is often encountered by both families and clinicians, is that the mental health system can be very individualistic in its view of symptoms and related treatments.

The clinician has a valuable role in providing psychoeducation to each family member so that they understand their "role" in the current family situation, while also understanding how they can help to change it. Supporting and educating families can be an effective tool in improving the functioning of the individual with the difficulties, as there is less conflict, blame and misunderstanding within the family system. The individual gains a great deal from intensive support and understanding of their circumstance and this impacts positively on their treatment and recovery (Henggeler, 1999). Transparency (i.e., the sharing of information and the process of treatment) between clinicians, young people, and families is crucial. The clinician's understanding of the individual's problems is shared with family members, who can otherwise complain of feeling neglected in the treatment. This then contributes to the family feeling an increasing sense of mastery as their understanding improves.

COLLABORATION/COERCION THEORY

The IMYOS model aims to use interventions and practices that respect and empower clients, promote collaboration and transparency, and move to equalizing client-client-clinician power. This set of principles clearly articulates key practice elements in establishing and maintaining collaboration. The current sections will begin by outlining the key elements of this theory and then discuss these as they are relevant to IMYOS.

Collaboration/Coercion Principles

The principles of collaboration/coercion guide the clinician in maintaining a collaborative relationship even when more coercive interventions are warranted (Bikerton, O'Brien, & Wallace, 2001). Dawson and Macmillan (1988), and Henggeler et al. (1999), would agree that coercive approaches in the care of young people/families are often unhelpful and unnecessary. The collaboration/coercion approach suggests that a collaborative relationship between clinician and young person incorporates a shared understanding of the problem. A willingness to work in partnership against the problem is seen as essential to collaboration (Bikerton et al., 2001). However, it is a reality in mental health that legislative frameworks may require more coercive interventions in times of crisis, such as when a young person is at high risk of suicide.

The collaboration/coercion approach promotes transparent communication when the clinician needs to move outside collaboration. If clinicians are able to overt the situation in which they may need to "intervene" in a more "coercive" manner, it is more likely that a collaborative relationship can be maintained overall. This framework suggests that there are clear situations that will likely mean a therapeutic relationship is less collaborative; when the clinician and client have (1) no agreement on the problem or the impact of the problem, (2) no willingness to work in partnership against the problem, and (3) client, community, or clinician safety is compromised. The principles suggest that it is in these situations a clinician might shift their role to a more "coercive" one in order to prioritise safety.

Implications for Intervention

In practice, a collaborative stance is necessary in interventions with the individual, family and system. Collaboration is fostered and cultivated by (1) transparency, (2) flexibility and creativity of approaches, and (3) joint participation.

Transparency. The clinician openly shares their understanding and concerns regarding the problem and informs the young person and their family of contact with and information gained from all sources. IMYOS stresses the importance of keeping the young person actively involved and informed of the process of assessment. The clinician openly discusses the safety framework (including theoretical, ethical, legal and organizational structures as appropriate) and invites the young person to co-create an individualized "safety plan." IMYOS also invites significant others (parent, carers, teachers, etc.) to be part of that plan. Where a young person refuses to participate a safety plan is drawn up using the information available and this is communicated in detail and in writing to the young person (e.g., when it will be enacted, by whom, why, and how). We routinely share our understanding of the young persons presentation (including the Safety Plan and assessment where possible) with the family and other professionals involved. IMYOS may hold joint family and/or professionals sessions that afford the opportunity for differences of opinion to be overted and acknowledged.

Flexibility and creativity of approaches. The IMYOS model allows interventions to incorporate individual, family and systemic work. It advocates approaches that are youth/family friendly, nonblaming and respectful (e.g., when to see the young person, where, and for how long, for what purpose). The young person and their family guide the interventions, if they are willing to participate. The clinician outlines her/his role, their conceptualisation of the young persons presentation and possible interventions. This includes clinicians explicitly stating what they can and can't do, and providing a rationale for the same, for instance that, successful work can only occur in a context in which both the client and clinician are safe.

Joint participation. The IMYOS clinician extends an invitation to a young person (and their family) to participate in the co-creation of how the young persons situation and difficulties are understood and the subsequent dialogue that forms part of the intervention. These dialogues aim to empower the young person and family, and are therefore made explicit and repeatedly renegotiated.

The principles of transparency, flexibility and joint participation as part of fostering a collaborative approach are echoed in our work with the system around young people. IMYOS clinicians explain their stance of transparency to all people involved with a young person and encourage them to follow suit (this is also modelled in meetings and day-to-day liaisons). IMYOS follow up situations where this has not occurred and attempts to discuss the situation in light of the goal of collaboration and transparency across the client-family-professional system. We have noticed that if we are finding a young person "difficult" it is probable that other professionals are also struggling in some way. It is likely that we are making incorrect assumptions about roles and actions of others without verification. This can affect the overall collaboration of the system and family, leading to conflict, splitting, and fragmentation that may compromise engagement and safety.

In our experience, providing a transparent and collaborative framework for the young person, family, and system results in a greater strength of relationship. By promoting trust as the basis of all therapeutic relationships, the possibility for ongoing collaborative work exists even when coercive approaches have been necessary. Experience suggests that people can better manage more coercive interventions if they feel that they have been forewarned.

RELATIONSHIP MANAGEMENT THEORY

Relationship management is one of the "relational stances" used by IMYOS. As with different elements of the IMYOS model, it should be noted that it is not possible (or advisable) to employ this approach with all young people, but IMYOS clinicians may draw on some of these principles. This section will summarize the principles of this perspective in relation to IMYOS work, and then discuss the implications of these for intervention.

Relationships Management Principles and IMYOS

Dawson and MacMillan (1993) describe the "relationship management" theory which aids our understanding of the problematic therapeutic relationships frequently experienced by and with these complex young people. Informed by work with individuals with Borderline Personality Disorder (BPD), the idea acknowledges that the mental health system has, at times, created very problematic relationships with some clients. The main principles include: (1) assumptions regarding the competency of the individual; (2) the use of process, not content, of therapeutic sessions; and (3) the formation of a corrective therapeutic relationship. The principles emphasize that it is important to do no harm, reduce chaos, and to moderate the often distorted relationship between the young person and the health care system. These principles highlight the need to maintain positive unconditional regard through remembering that young people are having legitimate experiences even if they appear "manipulative."

The essence of "relationship management" is about *not* rescuing a client, i.e., reasserting the competence of the individual. It assumes the client will eventually come to the solution themselves, although this may take time and involve the clinician sitting with the discomfort of relinquished control and possible risk as the client learns to manage themselves more adaptively. The clinician cannot enter into this approach of "relationship management" without the full support and acceptance of his/her institution.

"Relationship management" desires relationships which are empathic, respectful, collaborative and incorporate a clear, consistent and transparent treatment approach. This is particularly important in mental health where clinical rules afford a certain power.

The developmental stage of the young person needs to be thoroughly assessed to determine if "relationship management" is an appropriate approach. Although it has proven very powerful in empowering clients to learn to help themselves and offering a corrective relationship experience, careful consideration must be given to the cognitive and emotional developmental and environmental stages and chronological age of clients before proceeding. Discussion with team, supervisor, or managers can aid in deciding its clinical use.

Implications for Intervention

"Relationship management" proposes the idea of "no-therapy therapy," suggesting that being helpful is not always helpful. It is described as "less active assistance," offering the form of therapy without the content, thus allowing the young person to be responsible for his or her own care. The clinician would offer the client time limited regular meetings, providing an opportunity and structure for the young person to talk and the clinician to listen in a benign, neutral, yet warm manner. It is important that the "no-therapy" concept is not interpreted as being unavailable or rejecting, but rather less actively responding to the helping and problem solving behaviors the young person is often attempting to elicit from the clinician. To maintain the "no-therapy" relationship the clinician does not ask piercing questions, or offer advice, guidance, or interpretations, or enter into power and control situations/battles. The young person internalizes this as, "I am incompetent." Clinicians must assume the client comes to the process as a responsible and competent person, and overtly rescind the clinician's potentially powerful and controlling role.

IMYOS has also incorporated "relationship management" in family work. The principles are shared with family members to assist them to position themselves differently with their family member, possibly resulting in fewer control battles.

Psycho education, supervision, and consultation are fundamental in assisting clinicians who utilize a "relationship management" approach. The support of all workers is essential for this process to work. This may involve offering a supportive and reflective space for all professionals involved in the care of a young person, to develop a shared understanding of the treatment approach, and to acknowledge the inevitable difficulties encountered in working with these clients. It affords exploration of a professional's experience of control battles with young people, how they may respond differently and their self-efficacy to do so. When working with very complex young people we would *expect* difficulties to emerge between workers, and aim to create a space where these can be openly discussed. "Relationship management" appears to deny the expression of therapeutic qualities (such as empathy, helping and caring) that attract us to the work. It is Dawson and MacMillan's (1993) thesis that these very qualities cause harm to the borderline client and using the apparently less empathic relationship management approach ultimately provides better care and help. IMYOS has found that empathy can coexist with this approach (and arguably should), and it is perhaps the paternalistic notions of helping and caring which can be experienced as problematic.

CASE STUDY

The following case study illustrates how the different theories described above can be integrated in the treatment of IMYOS clients. The process of integration generally occurs on a case-by-case basis and is informed by the clients' presentation.

Lucy (name changed), 14 years of age, was referred to IMYOS with a 2 year history of polysubstance abuse, homicidal threats, self-harming behaviors, recurrent suicidal ideation and two previous attempts. She displayed oppositional behaviors, which resulted in her being expelled from numerous schools. It was reported that Lucy presented with promiscuous behaviors and that she had communication and learning difficulties.

Initial engagement was slow. The IMYOS clinician made repeated attempts to see Lucy, often finding her door unanswered. When Lucy was absent, letters and notes were left to document the clinician's persistent efforts to build a therapeutic relationship.

Family Work/Systems Theory

The IMYOS clinician visited Lucy's parents and her paternal grandmother (with Lucy's permission) to gain insight into Lucy's childhood and family background. The family assessment revealed that Lucy had witnessed domestic violence and had experienced severe intra-familial abuse. This gave the clinician insight into why Lucy may struggle to connect with others and use violence to cope with her persistent fear that others may reject and/or abuse her (Attachment Theory/Cognitive Analytic Therapy (CAT)).

The IMYOS clinician engaged Lucy's mother by listening to her and validating her role and experience in the family (Family Systems Theory).

This trust allowed the clinician to suggest different ways of responding to Lucy rather than continuing to reject and punish her.

The IMYOS clinician met with the child protection and drug and alcohol worker every fortnight to develop and implement a consistent approach and treatment plan. This allowed Lucy to feel more in control of herself because she knew how the people around her would respond as they were communicating and had a shared understanding.

A "safety plan" was created in collaboration with Lucy. The safety plan clearly documented roles and responsibilities in responding to Lucy when she was "in crisis" and outlined a framework of how to assist Lucy most effectively. The "safety plan" was given to all the professionals and family members involved in Lucy's care, allowing the system to feel contained and mutually supported (Systems Theory).

Individual Work

The main focus of individual work with Lucy was the development of a transparent and collaborative therapeutic relationship. On the basis of this relationship, the IMYOS clinician was able to provide Lucy with important feedback about the impact of her ways of communicating and behaving. For example, when Lucy became threatening towards the IMYOS clinician, she was reminded that her abusive behavior would result in the therapy session being terminated, which consequently may lead her to feeling rejected. By informing Lucy that the IMYOS clinician didn't intend to reject her, but at the same time was unable to tolerate her threats, Lucy became increasingly aware of the potential impact of her abusive behaviors on herself and others. At times Lucy would run off from a session following a discussion about her abusive manners, threatening to never see the clinician again, but she always returned within the same week.

During therapy Lucy gained insight into the association between her traumatic past and her recurrent destructive intra-and interpersonal patterns. (Attachment/Trauma Theory/CAT). Lucy often talked about how she felt "out of control" and that no one could possibly help contain her, thus leading to a greater sense of being out of control (CAT). Lucy's problematic interactional patterns were illustrated well by the pictorial and narrative aspect of CAT, which suited Lucy's learning style and developmental stage (Developmental Theory).

Lucy was regularly seen by the IMYOS psychiatrist who prescribed an antidepressant and a low dose of an atypical antipsychotic. This medication seemed to assist Lucy's mood and also helped her impulse control that had a great impact on her ability to tolerate therapy as well as reduce her aggressive behaviors.

Discharge

When Lucy was discharged from IMYOS after two and a half years she said that her relationship with the IMYOS worker had helped her engage because it had "clicked after some time" that the IMYOS clinician "was there" and had not been judgemental or rejecting. Lucy also said that the IMYOS clinician always explained to her all aspects of her treatment including a rationale for particular interventions. Lucy subjectively reported an improvement in her life. Possibly the greatest evidence of this is her effort to phone the IMYOS clinician on her 18th birthday and exclaim "I made it to eighteen," something she previously had not anticipated or wished for.

Lucy continues to have difficulties within her relationships but she manages her aggression much better. Lucy hasn't self-harmed for the last year of contact with IMYOS and has not attempted suicide within her episode of care. Lucy has reduced her substance use and has reconnected with her family.

IMYOS TEAM SUPPORTS

The integration of theories outlined in the IMYOS model applies not only to the work with young people, their families, and systems, but also to the functioning of the IMYOS team. The IMYOS team is an important part of the environment and many of the principles described above can be applied to the team. The team incorporates extensive support and safety practices that are considered essential to the provision of high quality service. These theories are applied to the teamwork and functioning via the leaderships in the team, modeling in interactions within the team and with other colleagues. For example, practice principles such as transparency, collaboration, and the establishment of safe relationships are overtly considered in team functioning. Additionally, attachment, trauma, and family systems theory aid the team to consider their responses to young people. A team undertaking such complex work requires opportunity to reflect on their work, just as they are asking their clients to do in their lives.

Leadership in the team can aim to model all of the above, specifically awareness of the power within relationships and its relatedness to trauma (vicarious), awareness of each member's, and the team's stage of development. Additionally, awareness of the functioning of the team is encouraged by the use of an external team (group) supervisor to allow reflection on the impact of the work on this system.

CONCLUDING COMMENTS

This model has developed from 7 years of clinical practice with high-risk, difficult-to-engage, complex-needs young people with mental health difficulties. Emerging evidence suggests that intensive outreach programs need to be multifaceted in their conceptualizations and interventions. The current model guides practical application integrating well-established theories. The IMYOS team aims to complete a procedural description of the work as well as an audit detailing the characteristics of the client group. Following these reports the team aims to undertake empirical research looking into the effect of IMYOS interventions.

NOTE

1. Refers to a person involved professionally in the care of an IMYOS client (who is not a mental health worker).

REFERENCES

American Psychiatric Association (1994). *Diagnostic and Statistical Manual of Mental Disorders* (4th Edition). American Psychiatric Association: Washington, DC.

Ackerman, N.W. (1966). *Treating the Troubled Family.* New York: Basic Books.

Beck, J.S. (1995). *Cognitive Therapy: Basics and Beyond.* New York: Guilford Press.

Bikerton, A., O'Brien, C., & Wallace, L. (2001). *Collaboration or coercion: Achieving balance in the care of high risk families.* Paper presented at Pan Pacific Family Therapy Congress, September 2001.

Blake, D.D., & Sonnenberg, R.T. (1998). Outcome research on behavioural and cognitive-behavioural treatments for trauma survivors. In V.M. Follette, J.I. Ruzek, & F.R. Abueg (Eds.), *Cognitive-behavioral therapies for trauma* (pp. 15–47). New York: Guilford Press.

Bowlby, J. (1979). *The Making and Breaking of Affectional Bonds.* London: Tavistock Publications.

Cicchetti, D., & Rogosch, F.A. (2002). A Developmental Psychopathology Perspective on Adolescence. *Journal of Consulting and Clinical Psychology, Vol. 70*, 6–20.

Davidson, L.M., Inslicht, S.S., & Baum, A. (2000). Traumatic stress and posttraumatic stress disorder among children and adolescents. In A.J. Sameroff, M. Lewis, & S.M. Miller (Eds), *Handbook of Developmental Psychopathology, Second Edition* (pp. 723–737). New York: Kluwer Academic/Plenum Publishers.

Dawson, D., & MacMillan, H. (1993). *Relationship management of the Borderline Patient: From Understanding to Treatment.* New York: Brunen/Mazel.

Dembo, J., & Schmeidler, J. (2002). *Family Empowerment Intervention. An Innovative Service for High-Risk Youth and Their Families.* New York: The Haworth Press.

Feldman, S.S., & Elliot, G.R. (Eds.). (1990). *At the Threshold: The developing adolescent.* Cambridge, MA: Harvard University Press.

Fergusson, D.M., Lynskey, M.T., & Horwood, L.J. (1996). Childhood sexual abuse and psychiatric disorder in young adulthood: I. Prevalence of sexual abuse and factors associated with sexual abuse. *Journal of the American Academy of Child and Adolescent Psychiatry, Vol. 35*, 1355–1364.

Golier, J., & Yehuda, R. (2002). Neuropsychological processes in post-traumatic disorder. *Psychiatric Clinics of North America, Vol. 25*, 295–315.

Henggler, S.W., Schoenwald, S.K., Borduin, C.M., Rowland, M.D., & Cunningham, P.B. (1998). *Multisystemic Treatment of Antisocial Behaviour in Children and Adolescents.* New York: The Guilford Press.

Henggeler, S.W., Rowland, M.D., Randall, J., Ward, D.M., Pickrel, S.G., Cunningham, P.B., Miller, S.L., Edwards, J., Zealberg, J.J., Hand, L.D., & Santos, A.B. (1999). Home-Based Multisystemic Therapy as an Alternative to the hospitalisation of Youths in Psychiatric Crisis: Clinical Outcomes. *Journal of the American Academy of Child & Adolescent Psychiatry, Vol. 38*, 1331–1339.

Holmbeck, G.N., & Updegrove, A.L. (1995). Clinical developmental interface: Implications of developmental research for adolescent psychotherapy. *Psychotherapy, Vol. 32*, 16–33.

Lanyado, M. (2001). Daring to try again: The hope and pain of forming new attachments. *Therapeutic Communities, Vol. 22*, 5–18.

Lewis, M. (Ed.). (1996). *Child and Adolescent Psychiatry: A comprehensive textbook.* Baltimore, MD: Williams & Wilkins.

Masten, A.S., & Coatsworth, J.D. (1998). The development of competence in favorable and unfavorable environments: Lessons from research on successful children. *American Psychologist, Vol. 53*, 205–220.

Minuchin, S. (1974). *Families and Family Therapy.* Cambridge, MA: Harvard University Press.

O'Donohue, W., Fanetti, M., & Elliott, A. (1998). Trauma in children. In V.M. Follette, J.I. Ruzek, & F.R. Abueg (Eds.), *Cognitive-behavioral therapies for trauma* (pp. 355–382). New York: Guilford Press.

Peterson, C. (1996) *Looking Forward Through the Lifespan. Developmental Psychology.* Hong Kong: Prentice Hall.

Pynoos, R.S., Steinberg, A.M., & Piacentini, J.C. (1999). A developmental psychopathology model of childhood traumatic stress and intersection with anxiety disorders. *Biological Psychiatry, Vol. 46*, 1542–1554.

Ryle, A., & Kerr, I. (2002). *Introducing Cognitive Analytic Therapy: principles and practice.* Chichester, UK: Wiley.

Schwartz, E.D., & Perry, B.D. (1994). The posttraumatic response in children and adolescents. *Psychiatric Clinics of North America, Vol. 17,* 311–326.

Shalev, A.Y. (1996). Stress versus traumatic stress: From acute homeostatic reactions to chronic psychopathology. In B.A. van der Kolk, A.C. McFarlane, & L. Weisaeth (Eds.), *Traumatic stress: The effects of overwhelming experience on mind, body, and society* (pp. 77–101). New York: Guilford Press.

Shepheris, C., Renfro-Michel, E., & Doggett, R. (2003). In-Home Treatment of Reactive Attachment Disorder in a Therapeutic Foster Care System: A Case Example. *Journal of Mental Health Counselling, Vol. 25,* 76–88.

Steinhauer, P.D., & Rae-Grant, Q. (Eds.). (1983). *Psychological Problems of Child in the Family. Second Edition, Revised Enlarged.* New York: Basic Books.

van der Kolk, B.A. (1996). The body keeps the score: Approaches to psychobiology of posttraumatic stress disorder. In B.A. van der Kolk, A.C. McFarlane, & L. Weisaeth (Eds.), *Traumatic stress: The effects of overwhelming experience on mind, body, and society* (pp. 214–241). New York: Guilford Press.

van der Kolk, B.A., & McFarlane, A.C. (1996). The black hole of trauma. In B.A. van der Kolk, A.C. McFarlane, & L. Weisaeth (Eds.), *Traumatic stress: The effects of overwhelming experience on mind, body, and society* (pp. 3–21). New York: Guilford Press.

Wagner, A.W., & Linehan, M.M. (1998). Dissociative behaviour. In V.M. Follette, J.I. Ruzek, & F.R. Abueg (Eds.), *Cognitive-behavioral therapies for trauma* (pp. 191–225). New York: Guilford Press.

White, M. (1990). *Narrative Means to Therapeutic Ends.* New York: W.W. Norton.

White, M. (2000). *Reflections on Narrative Practice.* Adelaide: Dulwich Centre Publications.

The Young Schema Questionnaire in Group Therapy: A Client-Focused Approach

Kathy Fitzsimmons, PhD, C Psych
Sheila Gallagher, MSW, RSW
Sandra Blayone, RN, BScN
Debbie Chan, MSW, RSW
Wendy Leaitch, Reg. OT (ONT)
Nancy Veals, RN, BScN
Nancy Wilkinson, PhD, C Psych

There is a paucity of program evaluation research of hospital-based group psychotherapy programs. Furthermore, most of the measurement is based on the quantity or intensity of psychiatric symptoms, such as level of depression or anxiety.

In hospital-based group programs, usually comprised of a chronically depressed and anxious population, there is a need to treat and measure underlying issues that lead to the symptoms of depression and anxiety. Over the course of therapy, clients may experience many significant changes which will affect the current intensity of symptoms, and will also affect some of the roots of psychological distress. In our treatment program, it was apparent that many people were discussing and changing relationships patterns, including one's view of oneself, view of others, and view of oneself in relation to others.

Young and Klosko's (1994) conceptualization of interpersonal schemas serves as a useful framework to identify and measure one's interpersonal issues that are addressed in psychotherapy. Researchers recognized that traditional cognitive-behavioral approaches were less effective with personality-disordered patients, and patients with treatment-resistant anxiety and depression (Young & Lindemann, 1992). Consequently, Young and Klosko (1994) placed a greater emphasis on childhood origins and core personal themes. They focused on "schemas," which are pervasive patterns or themes one has regarding one's self and relationship with others. Schemas develop in childhood and are elaborated and modified throughout one's life.

Young outlined maladaptive schemas that address unmet needs and self-defeating life patterns. The individual schemas fit into five clusters.

The *Disconnection or Rejection* cluster of schemas includes the expectation that one's basic needs for security, safety, or nurturance will not be met. *Impaired Autonomy or Performance* focuses on the expectation that one will not be able to function independently. A schema in the *Impaired Limits* cluster includes difficulty setting and meeting internal limits or meeting responsibilities to others. In contrast, *Other-directed-ness* involves the excessive focus on others, at the expense of one's own needs. *Overvigiliance and Inhibition* involves the suppression of emotions or choices, or rigid rules or expectations about behavior (Young, 2003).

The therapy provided in the current research is a 6-week, multidisciplinary, day treatment program designed to assist clients in making changes in self-concept and life patterns in order to alleviate symptoms of depression and anxiety. The Young Schema Questionnaire (Young & Brown, 1994) was used to help clients identify their personal issues. Clients were encouraged to explore how their schemas impacted daily functioning and relationships, and how schemas related to their symptoms of anxiety or depression. Cognitive-behavioral techniques were also used as a mechanism of change. Changes in the intensity of the schemas can be interpreted as a more global measure of functioning which may be indicative of long-lasting changes.

The nature of the current research was twofold. First, the goal was to identify how frequently clients presented with each schema. The second goal was to measure any changes in the maladaptive schemas during the course of treatment.

METHOD

Participants

The sample consisted of 92 consecutive adult clients (74 women, 18 men) who completed a mental health day treatment program in a general hospital setting. Hospital psychiatrists referred clients from the inpatient unit, the emergency walk-in crisis unit, and from outpatient psychiatry. Almost all clients presented with a mood and/or anxiety disorder. Concurrent substance abuse disorders, personality disorders, and suicidal ideation were also common. Exclusionary criteria included active psychosis, antisocial traits, and an inability to refrain from abusing substances during the group time. All clients voluntarily permitted the use of the data in their files for research purposes.

Materials

The Young Schema Questionnaire (short version) (Young & Brown, 1994) is comprised of 75 statements that a person might use to describe him/herself. Respondents are asked to read each statement and identify how well the statement currently describes them, using a 6-point scale. The wording of Young's original schemas was slightly modified in order to be more suitable for clients. This questionnaire identifies 15 schemas, which include: lack of emotional support, fear of abandonment, mistrust, social isolation, low self-esteem, failure to achieve (or disappointment in your accomplishments), dependence on others, fear of harm or illness, enmeshment with parents, subjugation, self-sacrifice, emotional inhibition, high expectations, entitlement, and insufficient self-discipline.

Adequate test re-test reliability for the schema subscales has been documented (average r =.76), and the subscales also show considerable internal consistency (average alpha =.90) (Schmidt, Joiner, Young, & Telch, 1995). There is also ample evidence of construct and divergent validity of the Young Schema Questionnaire with a variety of populations, including a psychiatric day treatment program (Welburn et al., 2002), university students (Schmidt et al., 1995), and counseling center outpatients (Glaser et al., 2002). In a psychiatric day treatment sample, similar to the one used in the current study, Welburn et al. (2002) found that all subscales, except for emotional deprivation, were correlated with symptoms of depression and/or anxiety. Multiple regression analysis also revealed that some subscales were predictors of anxiety, depression, or paranoia, further supporting the construct validity.

Procedure

Clients were asked to complete the Young Schema Questionnaire (Young & Brown, 1994) during the first orientation session to the program. Scores were then calculated and each client's highest scores (usually 1 to 4 schemas, depending on how the scores clustered) were selected. Written feedback was provided to clients during the second orientation session, describing each of their identified schemas that they had scored highest on. Clients were asked to review and interpret their scores during this session.

Following three orientation sessions, clients completed the 4-week active treatment phase of the program. All therapy was provided within a group format, and consisted of 2–3 group therapy sessions per day, 4 days per week. Treatment followed a cognitive-behavioral framework, and groups included psychotherapy, coping with relationship schemas, expressive therapy, skill development, mood management, communication, and self-esteem.

In the relationship schemas group, clients were encouraged to discuss their identified maladaptive schemas by relating their schemas to their day-to-day lives and to explore how their schemas may be related to the onset and maintenance of their depression and anxiety.

Clients discussed the origins of their schemas and how these experiences could be reframed. For example, being teased as a child may have contributed to low self-esteem and social isolation. As an adult, the client was encouraged to reframe their understanding of why they may have been teased. The group also focused on identifying and challenging the underlying beliefs and identifying behavior patterns that maintain the schemas. For example, if one believes they do not fit in with others, they are likely to avoid social situations and their avoidance would function to maintain the belief that they do not belong.

Following the 4-week treatment phase of the program, clients participated in two discharge groups in which they reviewed their treatment progress and completed the Schema Questionnaire again (Young & Brown, 1994). They were each provided with a written interpretation that outlined their pre and post schema scores. They were given the opportunity to review the information and discuss their reactions regarding changes to their schema scores.

RESULTS

Frequency of Schemas

Table 1 displays the percentage of clients who endorsed each schema. A tendency to be self-sacrificing in relationships was endorsed as a significant issue by more than half (54%) of the sample. The second most common schema was having high expectations (47%). It is interesting to note that there was relatively low endorsement of Enmeshment, Dependency, and Entitlement schemas.

TABLE 1. Percentage of clients endorsing each schema

Schema	Percentage
Self-sacrifice	54%
High Expectations	47%
Lack of Emotional Support	34%
Social Isolation	32%
Subjugation	23%
Fear of Abandonment	22%
Low Self Esteem	20%
Mistrust	18%
Failure to Achieve	16%
Insufficient Self-Discipline	15%
Emotional Inhibition	15%
Fear of Harm or Illness	12%
Enmeshment with Parents	9%
Dependence on Others	8%
Entitlement	5%

Pre–Post Differences in Schemas

A series of paired-samples t-tests revealed that there was a significant *decrease* in 8 of the 15 schemas at the end of treatment. The schemas that significantly decreased following treatment included: self-sacrifice, high expectations, social isolation, subjugation, fear of abandonment, low self esteem, mistrust, and entitlement. There was not a significant increase in any of the schemas following treatment. See Table 2 for t-scores and levels of significance.

DISCUSSION

Frequencies of Schemas

The tendency to be self-sacrificing in relationships was the most commonly endorsed schema. This is consistent with the most typical clinical presentation of clients in the day treatment program. The most typical pattern is characterized by a woman who has sacrificed her needs for her children and partner, and after years of not having her needs met, she has

TABLE 2. The mean differences between pre and post schema scores, standard deviations and t-test values

Schema	X difference in pre-post	SD	t-score
Self-Sacrifice	3.34	6.47	t(49) = 3.65***
High Expectations	2.84	6.30	t(42) = 2.92**
Social Isolation	4.97	6.43	t(28) = 4.16***
Subjugation	4.81	6.71	t(20) = 3.29**
Fear of Abandonment	6.65	7.52	t(19) = 3.96***
Low Self Esteem	8.33	8.25	t(17) = 4.28***
Mistrust	4.71	5.81	t(16) = 3.34**
Entitlement	7.40	2.30	t(4) = 7.19**
Lack of Emotional Support	8.06	6.07	t(30) = 0.74
Failure to Achieve	5.07	9.41	t(14) = 2.09
Insufficient Self-Discipline	3.86	8.31	t(13) = 1.74
Emotional Inhibition	3.43	5.25	t(13) = 2.44*
Fear of Harm or Illness	5.45	6.85	t(10) = 2.64*
Enmeshment with Parents	0.63	5.21	t(7) = 0.34
Dependence on Others	11.29	8.16	t(6) = 3.67

*= p < .05. **= p < .01. ***= p < .001.

been chronically depressed. Many clients identified life experiences, such as childhood neglect or assuming a parent-like role as a child, that had contributed to the development of a self-sacrificing schema. It should be noted that 80% of the sample was female, and although many males also report self-sacrificing in relationships, the results may have been different with a more balanced sample.

Anecdotally, in therapy most clients discussed a lack of emotional support during childhood, but only one third endorsed this as one of their most significant issues. It is likely that many clients have not had sufficient emotional support, but that the lack of emotional support has led to other maladaptive schemas that are more salient or more salient or more focused on the present. For example, someone who lacks emotional support may learn to be mistrustful of others or develop high expectations to gain support. Further, a history of poor emotional support may be manifest in current beliefs that one does not "fit in" socially (social isolation) or in low self esteem.

It is interesting to note that 54% of clients reported an interpersonally focused schema (e.g., self-sacrifice) and 47% reported an achievement-focused schema (e.g., high expectations). This is consistent with the literature outlining tow personality subtypes linked to vulnerability to depression. Both psychodynamic and cognitive theories of depression distinguish between two pathways to depression. The interpersonally focused pathway, labeled as "dependent" (Nietzel & Harris (1990), "anaclitic" (Blatt, 1974), and "socio-tropic" (Beck, 1983), is marked by an intense need for love and acceptance to maintain a fragile self-esteem, and consequently, depression may be pre-cipitated by a disruption in interpersonal relationships. In contrast, the achievement-focused pathway, also termed "achievement/autonomous" (Nietzel & Harris, 1990), "introjective" (Blatt, 1974), and "autonomous" (Beck, 1983), is characterized by a need to set and maintain high standards in order to maintain self-esteem. A failure to meet goals or expectations would result in self-criticism, guilt, and depression.

One factor that may influence the frequency of schemas is the attrition rate of the day treatment program. Approximately 62% of clients who begin the orientation process complete the program. Therefore, the reported frequencies are more descriptive of clients who complete the program, rather than those who enter or require treatment. Interpreted this way, it is logical that clients who sacrifice their own needs and have high expectations would have a greater commitment to the program. In contrast, clients lacking self-discipline or who perceived themselves as entitled are more likely to drop out of treatment.

Change in Schemas

Clients reported lower scores on approximately half of their schemas following treatment. A decrease in maladaptive schemas can be interpreted as support for the efficacy of the group treatment program. The goal of the treatment program is to help clients understand and begin to change the factors that lead to their depression or anxiety, including their view of self and relationships, and to experiment with different ways of coping. This research shows that clients made changes in the way they define themselves, by improving self-esteem, developing more realistic expectations of themselves, and importantly, learning to prevent self-criticism when they do not meet their expectations.

The group format provides an excellent forum to intensely challenge the interpersonal schemas. The very nature of a supportive group therapy process facilitates change in social isolation, fear of abandonment, and difficulty trusting others. Some items on the schema questionnaire that decreased following treatment included "I don't fit in" and "I feel that people will take advantage of me." During treatment, clients were openly encouraged to challenge themselves to share their experiences and emotions in groups and to experiment with trusting group members. As a result, they experienced support and acceptance and began to challenge the assumption that "everyone" will betray, criticize, or abandon them.

Clients also explored how subjugating their thoughts and emotions and being self-sacrificing contributed to relational problems, including not getting one's needs met. Some schema items that changed following treatment included "I think that if I do what I want I am only asking for trouble," and "I am a good person because I think of others more than myself." Clients explored how early experiences led to distorted perceptions of their value in relationships and expectations that people would be unwilling to meet their needs. They also discussed more appropriate roles for themselves in relationships and experimented playing different roles with others. Significant changes in the subjugation and self-sacrifice schemas suggest that clients began to make changes in their expectations of themselves and others in relationships.

A major focus of treatment is the development of coping skills. This includes coping with anxiety by working on distorted interpretations of situations, asking for help, and problem solving, i.e., determining, what one would do if something bad were to happen. The goal is to help clients move past the anticipatory anxiety, to re-evaluate the situation and feel empowered to cope with the "what if" scenario. Following treatment, there is evidence that clients felt less vulnerable, as demonstrated by lower fear of harm or illness schema scores, and increased comfort expressing their emotions to others to cope.

However, it is also possible that the decrease in some scores may have been influenced by the general decrease in distress levels after the treatment. That is, when one is feeling less depressed, they may see their issues (e.g., low self esteem) as less severe.

It may be surprising that no schemas increased as a result of treatment. Often a goal of therapy is to help clients to become more aware of issues or maladaptive patterns in their lives. One possible explanation for this may be that the chronic population served may already be aware of their issues. Alternatively, it may be that over the course of treatment, clients gained awareness but also worked on resolving these issues.

Client scores on approximately half of the schemas did not change following treatment. This may be due to small group sizes for some schemas, which interfered with statistical power. However, one schema with sufficient statistical power, lack of emotional support, did not change. It may be that some schemas are either less likely or more difficult to change. A lack of emotional support is largely influenced by past relationships. Treatment does not intend to alter one's perceptions of history, but rather attempts to help the client to cope and interpret these experiences in a less self-defeating manner. Treatment is focused more on how one may have been affected by a lack of emotional support, rather than focusing on the lack of emotional support itself.

Implications for Therapy

Client feedback indicated that the schema conceptualization helped them to feel understood and validated and helped them to gain insight into life changes that they could address during treatment. The labeling of issues in succinct and concrete terms allowed clients to relate their histories to present functioning without preoccupation with historical details. For example, a client's history of abuse could be related to issues of lack of emotional support and trust. These descriptors allow the client to focus on his/her current situation and help him/her to make connections between past experiences and current relationships as well as expectations of others. It also provides a focus of change. Clients can not change their abuse histories, but can make changes to current relational patterns that may have arisen from an abusive past.

Our results suggest that short-term group therapy does make significant changes in some schemas. This research supports the use of schemas as a richer, more detailed tool for program evaluation, which can supplement data on whether symptoms of depression and anxiety decrease over the course of treatment. The next step for the use of schemas as a measure of program evaluation would be to examine whether these changes in schemas persist over time, following treatment.

REFERENCES

Beck, A. T. (1983). Cognitive therapy of depression: New perspectives. In P.J. Clayton & J.E. Barrett (Eds.), *Treatment of depression: Old controversies and new approaches* (p. 265–290). New York: Raven Press.

Blatt, S. J. (1974). Levels of object representation in anaclitic and introjective depression. *The Psychoanalytic Study of the Child, 24,* 107–157.

Glaser, B. A., Campbell, L. F., Calhoun, G. B., Bates, J. M., & Petrocelli, J. V. (2002). The Early Maladaptive Schema questionnaire-short form: A construct validity study. *Measurement and Evaluation in Counseling Development, 35,* 2–13.

Nietzel, M. T., & Harris, M. J. (1990). Relationship of dependence and achievement/autonomy to depression. *Clinical Psychology Review, 10,* 279–297.

Schmidt, N. R., Joiner, T. E., Young, J., & Telch, M. J. (1995). The Schema Questionnaire: Investigation of psychometric properties and the hierarchical structure of a measure of maladaptive schemas. *Cognitive Therapy and Research, 19*(3), 295–321.

Welburn, K., Coristine, M., Dagg, P., Pontefract, A., & Jordan, S. (2002). The Schema Questionnaire-Short form: Factor analysis and relationship between schemas and symptoms. *Cognitive Therapy and Research, 26*(4), 519–530.

Young, J. (2003). *Early Maladaptive Schemas.* (Available from the Cognitive Therapy Centre, 36 West 44th Street, Suite 1007, New York, New York 10036)

Young, J., & Brown, G. (1994). *The Young Schema Questionnaire—Short Form.* (Available from the Cognitive Therapy Centre, 36 West 44th Street, Suite 1007, New York, New York 10036)

Young, J., & Klosko, J. (1994). *Reinventing your life: How to break free from negative life patterns and feel good again.* New York: Plume.

Young, J., & Lindemann, M. (1994). (1992). An integrative schema-focused model for personality disorders. *Journal of Cognitive Psychotherapy, 6,* 11–23.

SECTION 2: VIOLENCE, TRAUMA, AND RESILIENCE

Responding to the Individual Trauma of Domestic Violence: Challenges for Mental Health Professionals

Catherine Humphreys, PhD

To hold traumatic reality in consciousness requires a social context that affirms and protects the victim and that joins victim and witness in common alliance. For the individual victim, this social context is created by relationships with friends, lovers and family. For the larger society, the social context is created by political movements that give voice to the disempowered (Herman, 1992, p.9).

The arena of domestic violence intervention is changing. Particularly in those countries where there has been 25–30 years of experience in responding to the needs of women and children who have experienced domestic violence, significant shifts are occurring. While some aspects of domestic violence provision remain depressingly familiar, it is the changing areas (or even the potentially changing areas) of service provision and intervention that are the subject of this chapter, and I focus specifically on both the opportunities and threats of taking these issues forward in the mental health sector.

The quote from Judith Herman is used to highlight issues that are central to domestic violence intervention and that present challenges to health professionals who are more familiar with the "individual patient" focus of their practice. It is this tension between a medical model and a more holistic domestic violence intervention model which was both a theme in some of the papers and workshops at the 4th International Conference on Social Work in Health and Mental Health, and which also provides the focus for this article.

BACKGROUND

The impetus for exploring this area comes from research undertaken with domestic violence survivors whose experiences highlight both the strength and shortcomings of the responses to the emotional trauma that many reported. The research was funded by Women's Aid, England, the key organization that supports domestic violence survivors in the UK. Twelve outreach project (nonrefuge services) provided the research sites.

Women research participants were contacted via these services. Question-naires were distributed by project coordinators who assisted women with experiences of domestic violence to complete the questionnaires. In all, 180 questionnaire returns were received, which represented a return rate of 80%. A further 20 in-depth interviews were conducted, of whom four were with black and minority ethnic women. The findings from both the questionnaire and interviews showed that for this group of women using domestic violence outreach centers in the UK, experiences of physical trauma, emotional trauma, depression, and suicide attempts were perva-sive (Humphreys & Thiara, 2002).

When asked about their reasons for leaving the relationship, 60% of women said that they "feared for their mental health." This research undertaken in the UK supports the evidence from other studies that all point to very high rates of depression, posttraumatic stress, suicide, and self-harm in women experiencing domestic violence and other forms of abuse.[1] A brief overview of this literature is given to contextualize the issue.

A number of research overviews in the US (Golding, 1999; Cascardi, O'Leary, & Shlee, 1999; Jones, Highes, & Unterstaller, 2001) and in Australia (Taft, 2003) have helpfully bought together the research evidence in the area. Across 17 different studies, Golding (1999) found an average prevalence rate of depression amongst abused women of 47.6%, while the overview of studies by Cascardi et al. (1999) found rates from 38% to 83%. This incidence greatly exceeds that for women in the general population rated at about 10%. Cascardi et al. (1999) suggest that depression is a function of the attacks on the woman's sense of self.

A compounding issue for many women is the undermining of their sense of safety, which can lead to experiences of trauma. Women in the outreach center study spoke of panic attacks, high anxiety, and hypervigi-lance. An overview by Jones et al. (2001) of 42 studies found worryingly high rates of posttraumatic stress disorder (PTSD) similar to those found by Golding (1999) and Cascardi et al. (1999) in their overviews of 11 studies. These rates varied from 31% to 84% (Gleason, 1993; Kemp, Green, Hovanitz, & Rawlings, 1995) depending on the site from which the sample was drawn. Not surprisingly, women in refuges showed a higher rate of PTSD than those drawn from community based services (Kemp et al., 1995; Saunders, 1994).

Many of the women also spoke of feeling trapped and caged by the abuser's strategies of control. Stark and Flitcraft (1995) have argued that it is this sense of entrapment that will often lead women to attempt suicide. Many of the women's stories trace the increasingly extreme ways in which men tried to control their partners through these forms of "intimate terrorism" (Johnson & Ferraro, 2000), sometimes not even allowing them to go to the toilet alone.

Golding (1999) had also undertaken an overview of 13 studies of suicide and domestic violence. These studies again point to significantly heightened rates of suicide attempts among women who have been the subject of domestic violence. Rates vary considerably between research settings. A study by Stark and Flitcraft (1995) found that of 176 women identified through medical records at an accident and emergency service that 52 (30%) had been the subject of domestic violence during the sample year.

For black women in the US studies, the rate was considerably higher than for white women, featuring in 48.8% of the suicide attempts as against a rate of 22.2% for white women (Stark and Flitcraft, 1995). This is an issue which is now consistently noted into the UK. There are now some very important studies of elevated rates of self harm among Asian women under 30 (Merrill and Owens, 1986; Yazdani, 1998; Soni-Raleigh, 1996; Bhugra, 1999). The qualitative study by Yazdani, "Young Asian Women and Self-Harm," suggests that domestic violence, of which forced marriage was one aspect, was a factor for many, though not all, of the young Asian women.

In summary, the research evidence consistently points to the ways in which women's mental health and well-being is eroded by their experiences of living with domestic violence. Such findings are hardly surprising when the ways in which power and control are established over another person are considered. As one of the women in the outreach center study put so eloquently:

> I don't call it mental health, I call it symptoms of abuse. (Elaine, white British woman)

WOMEN'S EXPERIENCES OF THE MENTAL HEALTH SYSTEM

However, women's experiences of health and medical services were extremely varied. In relation to their mental health problems, these ranged from the neutral to the destructive (Humphreys & Thiara, 2003). Women first highlighted the fact that unless they had a "serious and enduring" mental illness, they were not considered the domain of mental health professionals. At times, there was a positive aspect to this exclusion.

> He (psychiatrist), said, I've one question for you Mrs X', and I said, 'What's that?'. He said, 'Why are you here and not your husband?' And I knew that I was normal . . . I should say . . . that there was no follow up of anything . . . . that was it really (Jenny).

So, while the psychiatrist quite rightly placed the responsibility for her problems onto her abusive husband, he did not provide her with an appropriate referral to services that might have assisted her to find safety or which acknowledged her considerable emotional distress. In effect, this psychiatrist saw no role for himself (or others) in responding to the trauma and depression she experienced as a result of the violence and abuse she had experienced.

The second problem for women accessing the mental health system was the lack of attention to domestic violence. The woman's depression, personality disorder, or suicidal tendencies become the focus of intervention and in this process the abuser and the results of his abuse become invisible.

> '. . . . I am irritated to this day that the people around me, that is, the health visitor, my social worker, his social worker, the GPs, in a way, all be it unwittingly, they perpetuated that myth in my head, because nobody else (until the domestic violence outreach worker) used the word 'violence'. . . (Lisa who met her ex-husband in a psychiatric hospital).

The lack of recognition and acknowledgement of the women's experiences of abuse can lead to an inadvertent collusion with the abuser. His accusation that she is "mad," "crazy," and "out of touch with reality" are given validation by mental health professionals who fail to ask about domestic violence and, if they do, may also minimize the connection with the women's symptoms and ongoing safety issues. In effect, the women's mental health treatment is separated from her abuse experiences.

Third, and at its worst, women experienced quite overt victim blaming from mental health or health professionals.

> The hospital was absolutely disgusting. I went in during the split. I took an overdose, because he was constantly on the phone, I couldn't take it anymore. They treated me terribly . . . . I did hear a couple (medical staff) in the corridor saying 'There's an OD case,

domestic violence. She's been in before, just leave her. She'll be out by morning'. I did get a leaflet given to me for something on housing (Kim).

Such experiences, which were noted by several women in the study, are parallel to the complaints about the minimization by police denoted by the term, "just a domestic." Stark and Flitcraft (1996) have carefully traced the process through which women admitted to A&E departments with injuries from the abuser or suicide attempts may initially (though not always) be treated sympathetically. However, after several admissions the woman becomes labelled as suffering mental health problems, often depression, "personality disorder," or "borderline personality disorder." Paradoxically, the control exerted by the abuser over the woman, particularly evident in her continuing to live with him, becomes seen as a symptom and indicator of the woman's mental health problems rather than the source of these problems.

Fourth, women's experiences of the mental health system are far from neutral. The stigmatizing aspects of being diagnosed with a mental health problem, whether that be depression, PTSD, or personality disorder can be experienced as profoundly disabling, particularly when they play into the abuser's psychological abuse that often takes the form of accusing her of being mad or crazy. These "flow-on effects" disable rather than empower the victimized woman. Particularly in child contact cases and in child protection proceedings, the slippage from a focus on the man's violence and abuse to the women's mental health problems can be profoundly damaging (Stanley & Penhale, 1999; Humphreys & Harrison, 2003) and distort the assessment of both the woman and the children's needs.

Taken together, from the women's perspective, contact with the mental health system has the potential to be either inadequate or damaging when the effects of violence and abuse are minimized or rendered invisible. Such damaging experiences have led some advocates to recommend "giving up on the mental health system" (Burstow, 2003), condemning it as an additional form of patriarchal violence (Chesler, 1972), which compounds rather than alleviates the abuse that women have suffered. Others, however, point to the number of women who are languishing inappropriately within the mental health system and the secondary abuse that this involves when practices more sensitive to their abusive experiences are undeveloped (Hager, 2004). Within the Quebec conference, a number of papers and workshops explored and problematized this complex relationship between women's abuse experiences and medical and health professionals (Palley, 2004; Dewees, Pulliam, & Roche, 2004) raising questions about how bridges may be built so that women's experiences of abuse are neither ignored nor pathologized.

FURTHER CONCERNS ABOUT THE MEDICAL MODEL

The issues raised by women highlight longstanding debates within the broad movement to support survivors of abuse that have often, though not solely, been articulated by women identified with the feminist movement.

Clearly, there are some issues raised by the women in the study which remain longstanding and depressingly familiar. The problems of violence and abuse remaining secret, unacknowledged, and hidden continue, and clearly survivors are still reporting being blamed as if they were complicit in their own abuse. Appropriate resources to respond to women's emotional needs in the aftermath of abuse remain inadequate. In the UK, there are limited counselling or support groups for women to access. This remains particularly the case for black and minority women (Bughra, 1999). These issues are exemplified in the outreach center study (Humphreys & Thiara, 2002). Black and minority women showed the same level of overwhelming problems as white women in the immediate post-separation period. However, when questioned about their experiences 6 months after separation, many white, British women were able to show a very marked improvement in their circumstances in relation to financial problems, their children's emotional and behavioral problems, and post-separation violence. The same could not be said for the majority of black and minority ethnic women. Statistically significant differences in their post-separation experiences emerged after 6 months, indicating that the path for these women was much more complex and difficult. Such evidence highlights the need for specialist services for black and minority ethnic women to address their complex needs.

There are also new emerging issues, not all of which were highlighted by the women in our study. These have come to light as the dissemination and implementation processes associated with this and other projects have developed (Carter, 2003) and the interviews with workers and advocates associated with outreach project have been analyzed.

First, there is the interesting issue of *mainstreaming*. This is the process through which previously marginalized problems and interventions move from being on the periphery of the policy and practice agenda, to recognition within the mainstream of statutory services such as the police, health, and child protection services. Fraser (1989) refers to this shift from "needs talk" among those directly affected by an issue, to the resourcing of needs through mainstream institutional sites, as a significant aspect of the "politics of need interpretation." A resulting issue is that domestic violence concerns then move into the remit of those who may not have the specialist knowledge or the experience of working in this area.

Some problems arise, of course, in arguing on the one hand that domestic violence remains underresourced and invisible, while on the other hand being dismayed at the inadequacy of responses when the issue moves into "the mainstream." On the surface this appears contradictory. However, it would also be problematic to not acknowledge some significant changes even if these may fall short of expectations. In the UK, there are now a raft of new domestic violence policies covering every government department (police, prosecution, health services, housing, child protection and family support services) as well as interdepartmental committees and interdepartmental ministerial committees. There has been an increase in funding in some areas. New legislation is being bought forward and at local level numerous domestic violence multi-agency forums and partnerships work proactively to develop services and policies to respond to the needs of domestic violence survivors and their children and challenge and intervene with perpetrators. The British Medical Association has bought out guidelines for its professionals and virtually every health specialty in nursing and medicine has a policy on domestic violence.

Relevant to this chapter, is the shift in the UK to acknowledging domestic violence as a serious threat to mental health encapsulated in the new mental health guidance, "Women into the Mainstream" (Department of Health, 2003). This document, issued by the Department of Health, acknowledges for the first time the profound effects of domestic violence on women's mental health. There remains, of course, the problem of implementation. New documents on mental health published since do not acknowledge violence and abuse as contributory factors to women's mental health, new inspection standards fail to recognize the implications of this policy document, and the associated budget for implementation is extremely limited. Nevertheless, the policy represents an important acknowledgement of the gendered nature of mental health problems and women's specific vulnerabilities.

A second issue is that of the *professionalization* of the response to domestic violence. Mental health problems are seen as the domain of professional intervention. Diagnosis and treatment, whether this is drug-based intervention or counseling, are seen to require specialist skills specific to professionals in medicine, psychology, and social work. In the US, the trauma counseling industry is now thriving, with clinical psychologists in the ascendancy. The prescribing of antidepressants and antianxiety drugs is at unprecedented levels, and a significant proportion of the women in refuges are using prescribed medication (Barron, 2004). In this process, the value of experience and the healing aspects of mutual support, long valued in domestic violence intervention, may be overshadowed.

The third aspect of this intervention is that the response is usually *individually* based. Doctors, psychiatrists, and other professionals typically hold individual consultations. A raft of different models have also been developed to respond to posttraumatic stress, including cognitive behavioral techniques (Herbert and Wetmore, 1999; Resick and Jordan, 1988), critical stress debriefing (Mitchell, 1983), eye movement desensitization reprocessing (EMDR) (Shapiro, 1989; 1995), and psychodynamic therapy (Lindy, 1996; Marmar, Weiss, & Pynoos, 1995). Whatever the approach, the effect has been to highlight the professional and specialist nature of intervention. Therapy has been overwhelmingly individually based and works very specifically to relieve the symptoms which create such significant distress for trauma survivors, including domestic violence survivors. Papers at the Quebec international conference by Jude Irwin and Lindsey Napier (2004) on mental health and domestic violence that looked more holistically at women's needs were welcome reminders that mental health work that works with survivors of trauma does not need to be dominated by practices primarily drawn from medicine or clinical psychology.

THIRTY YEARS OF EXPERIENCE

In the UK and other Western countries, women's services in the voluntary sector have had 30 years of experience in working with domestic violence survivors, including their children. The first women's refuge was established in London in the mid-70s. The majority of the women using refuges, helplines, and outreach programs are traumatized and often depressed, and a significant proportion have had suicide attempts (Humphreys & Thiara, 2003; Barron, 2004). There have been strategies developed which, while sometimes in need of updating, have been tested and positively evaluated by survivors over many years. Consistently, women say the same things about what makes a difference to their emotional recovery: lifting the blame and being helped to name the abuse; attention to their safety; being believed; a nonjudgemental approach; time, support and information; the ability to respond to multiple abuse experiences; and accessible services available outside standard working hours (Humphreys and Thiara, 2002). While many women have further specialist needs, these are foundational elements which are essential to any response to the woman's emotional well-being and that have often been provided by women working in the voluntary sector. Health services in the mainstream of provision need to question whether they can provide these basic elements that create the context through which recovery can occur.

It is now timely to return to the quote by Judith Herman used at the beginning of the chapter, as her writing highlights the areas which should form part of the backbone of work with survivors. Herman's seminal book, *Trauma and Recovery* (1992), explored overarching principles in the work with abuse survivors which recognized and normalized their experiences of trauma. Her work is particularly applicable to abuse survivors in the mental health system who she felt were too readily diagnosed with the spurious and unhelpful categories of borderline personality disorder, which detached their emotional pain from their experiences of abuse. She believed that posttraumatic stress was a more accurate description of their experiences, which opened the door to appropriate intervention connecting their abuse experiences to the way they were feeling and behaving.

Her work is of particular importance, as aspects of her approach could go some way to creating bridges between appropriate mental health services (particularly where women are inpatients as this was where Herman's work was based) and women's services. While her approach is that of a specialist professional, and many women have questioned the helpfulness of a new category of diagnosis (Berg, 2002; Burstow, 2003), she also emphasises the essential nature of re-establishing the woman's relationship network (connectivity) and the significance of situating individual work within its political context through social movements to support survivors. These are two core concepts that women's services in the voluntary sector have always emphasized—the notion of mutual self-help (women helping other women on the basis of their shared experiences) and the recognition that domestic violence and violence against women more generally are primarily social and political problems in which individual women and children are harmed.

These two issues are raised as they represent aspects of the intervention to support abuse survivors which are most at risk if the work of women's services becomes subsumed within standardized mental health and medical responses. The international conference held in Quebec for health and mental health social workers was a case in point. Many of the papers, particularly those on posttraumatic stress by social workers, discussed service provision and the work with trauma survivors reified from these broader contextual issues.

THE ROLE OF SOCIAL SUPPORT

A central aspect of establishing power and control over another person involves isolating them from as many people as possible, other than the perpetrator. Reconnecting women with other people, including their children, other women, and sympathetic family and friends is therefore a crucial element in recovery. For black and minority ethnic women for whom extended family and community relationships may be central to their identity, such reconnections may be particularly complex when, the perpetrator, supported by cultural norms, has "groomed" the family and community against her (Batsleer et al., 2002).

A group of research studies show in different ways that survivors of trauma and depression are assisted by supportive rather than critical or hostile relationships with family members and partners (Coker et al., 2002; Tarrier, Sommerfield, & Pilgrim, 1999). Resick (2001) provides an overview of research on the relationship between social support and PTSD. While highlighting the complexity of this concept, her overview provides compelling evidence that survivors of trauma with high social support had significantly lower rates of PTSD than those with poor support (Boscarino, 1995; Davidson, Hughes, Blazer, & George, 1991). More recent studies, however, have also suggested that the findings on social support may be gendered, with women responding particularly strongly to negative responses from family and friends (Andrews, Brewin, & Rose, 2003).

While, this research and the work by Herman (1992) on "connectivity" indicate that social support is a significant factor in recovery or buffering against the development of PTSD, the popularization of individual trauma counseling has let these aspects of trauma intervention become marginalized. The attention to the skills involved in supporting the development of social networks which has been a feature of relationship counselling (Laing, 2001; Sanders, 1992), has not been a prominent aspect of trauma intervention.

Similarly, while support groups are clearly seen to have a place in intervention to support survivors (Laing, 2001; Flannery, Irwin, & Copes, 2000), this aspect of the work in relation to posttraumatic stress has been given little attention relative to the discussion and development of EMDR, critical incident debriefing, and cognitive behavioral therapy.

SOCIAL MOVEMENTS

It would appear that while the role of social support has had minimal development within posttraumatic stress intervention and managing depression, the aspect of the discourse that has been most marginalized by the professionalized responses of clinical psychology and mental health professionals has been the significant role that social movements have to play in creating the social context through which survivors can find a space for affirmation and justice. While for some trauma victims this may not be an issue, in the arena of violence against women, where the context of the traumatic event/s involve shame, humiliation, and often criminal acts of violence against a background of a chronic social problem, the role of a supportive social movement has particular significance.

Social movements can be defined as organized efforts to promote or resist change in society that rely, at least in part, on noninstitutionalized forms of political action (Marx and McAdam, 1994). An aspect of the "new social movements" instigated in the 70s, and continuing in different forms to the present day, is the attention to social justice and the challenge to oppression and the processes of discrimination (Thompson, 2002). These are pivotal issues for abuse survivors where it can be argued that there is a widespread tendency for denial and minimization to dominate and subjugate stories of abuse and violence, particularly when they disrupt and undermine strongly held beliefs about social institutions such as the family (Herman, 1992). Providing an alternative discourse which validates the survivor's experience, recognizes her right to justice, and recasts the shame and humiliation of the abuse experience into a story that affirms her strength and resilience in the face of a violence, it could be argued, is an essential, though not necessarily measurable, role of the movements that support abuse survivors.

In the UK, it is difficult to point to an overarching women's movement. In fact it can be argued that there is a weakening of grassroots social movements, including the women's movement, which initially provided the platform from which support for the survivors of abuse originally occurred (Charles, 2000). At another level, developments within contemporary social movements recognize the significance of small, diverse localized actions and organizations rather than a unified body as the way in which social action and change occurs. It may be now more appropriate to point to the "network of organisations" (Melucci, 1989) which support survivors. These constitute a more diverse social movement than that previously associated with the women's movement.

In the UK, there remains an effective umbrella organization for women's refuges provided by the Women's Aid Federations of England, Wales, Scotland, and Northern Ireland. These organizations share a number of common principles in their work with survivors which provide the platform for political lobbying. These values include: a strong belief in mutual self help; a strengths-based approach to intervention; a commitment to advocacy; acknowledgement that women's individual stories are part of a wider social context in which violence against women is an endemic pattern; and a commitment to involving survivors in the organization of services (Hague, Mullender, & Aris, 2003). Historically, ideas have been drawn from radical feminism. Many other groups have now emerged, particularly among black and minority ethnic women (Southall Black Sisters and IMKAAN) and children's organizations (NSPCC, Barnardos, NCH Action for Children, and Childline) to articulate the specific needs of the women and children they represent. Alliances are then frequently made across these organizations to work together on particular social and political issues.

However, there is also a changing face to the movement to support survivors coming from two different directions. In this construction of social movements, the support for survivors has seen a potential widening of its base. Firstly, the service user movement for mental health survivors as well as abuse survivors is developing its own impetus. It is the former rather than the latter which is currently seeing the greatest development. Policy guidelines within the mental health arena (Dept of Health, 2003; Department of Health, 1999) quite explicitly recommend service user involvement in service developments, and some inspection regimes look for evidence of this dimension within their reviews. Mental health user forums are being established throughout the country and provide an alternative voice within the dominant, medicalized agenda (Wilson & Beresford, 2000). The strengthening of this base can provide opportunities for a more sympathetic and sensitive response to women abuse survivors.

In the UK, the mainstreaming of concern for domestic violence survivors has seen a wider group of professionals and organizations from both the statutory and voluntary sector involving themselves in more than 250 interagency forums across the country (Hague, Malos, & Dear, 1996). Many of these have now been transformed into active inter-agency groups against domestic violence with accountability within the broader but local, Crime and Disorder Reduction Partnerships.

While the representation of survivors of abuse may not be strong within these partnerships (Hague et al., 2003), and they are undoubtedly more conservative than the radical movement established by the second wave of feminism, they nevertheless often provide a commitment to keeping domestic violence (in particular) on the public agenda. This may not be "the voice" or the social movement that Herman (1992) might have originally envisaged; however, many of these partnerships are providing a very active and vocal local response to domestic violence with commitments to the crime and justice agenda as well as increasing the resources to survivors and some prevention programs in schools. They are therefore not organizations that should be ignored in a discussion of the public face of the movement to support survivors. They generally complement rather than contradict the work of the voluntary sector lobby groups striving to keep the needs of survivors on the social and political agenda.

An aspect of these more professionally based forums is that they are more accessible to a wide range of people now working in the area of domestic violence intervention. They therefore open up a *possibility* for wider engagement of mental health professionals with the broader movement to support survivors. However, to date, mental health services, particularly psychiatrists and psychologists, are rarely represented at these forums. Until this shift occurs, the disjuncture between mental health services and the social movements and organizations that give "voice to the disempowered" will remain, in spite of a potentially more inclusive (and more conservative) social movement to support survivors of abuse.

CONCLUSION

Domestic violence is a social problem, but one in which individual women, children, and some men also bear the emotional consequences. As work with individual survivors develops, it would seem that the importance of the social movement becomes greater rather than diminished, if the balance between the individual and the social is to be maintained.

Herman (1992) argued that just as an individual survivor of violence needs to both speak of the abuse and simultaneously deny what has happened, there are parallel processes within the social context. The need for a community or a culture to deny the presence of violence and abuse runs alongside the need to collectively acknowledge these destructive aspects of the society, if collusion and denial and, hence, abuse are not to continue. Particularly where the perpetrators of violence are powerful and influential, the ability to silence, shame, and discredit the traumatic reality of their victims can too easily gain ascendancy. This of course is most easily done through calling your victim "mad," pointing to their mental health problems and the vulnerability of their grip on reality. We are not in neutral territory when we explore the connections between mental health and domestic violence.

The challenge for individual health professions is recognizing the need and then finding the political commitment to participate in the wider agenda to support survivors. The challenge for the ever-changing face of the social movement to support survivors is how to find the spaces and the structures to include health professionals. These shifts can change the very nature of the social movement. Nevertheless, the attention to the development of social support and the movement to support survivors are central and not marginal aspects of an effective and meaningful response in the domestic violence arena. Fostering these aspects of the work needs to be the responsibility of every profession working in the area and part of keeping alive the energy, enthusiasm, and commitment which has characterized the diverse range of women, practitioners, policy makers, and researchers who have always contributed to ensuring that the voice of individual survivors is part of a wider agenda to stop domestic abuse.

NOTE

1. As the study was based in women's services I use the feminine form when speaking of domestic violence survivors while recognizing that while this is the dominant pattern, men are also at times abused both by other men and by their female partners.

REFERENCES

Andrews, B., Brewin, C., & Rose, S. (2003). Gender, social support and PTSD in victims of violent crime. *Journal of Traumatic Stress, 16* (4), 421–427.
Barron, J. (2004). Struggle to survive: Challenges for delivering services on mental health, substance misuse and domestic violence. Bristol: Women's Aid Publications.

Batsleer, J., Burnman, E., Chantler, K., McIntosh, H., Pantling, K., Smailes, S., & Warner, S. (2002). Domestic violence and minoritisation: Supporting women to independence. Manchester: Women's Studies Research Centre, Manchester Metropolitan University.

Berg, S. (2002). The PTSD diagnosis: Is it good for women? *Affilia, 17,* 55–68.

Bhugra, D., Desai, M., & Baldwin, D. (1999). Attempted suicide in west London, rates across ethnic communities. *Psychological Medicine, 29,* 1125–1130.

Boscarino, J. (1995). Post-traumatic stress and associated disorders among Vietnam veterans: The Significance of combat exposure and social support. *Journal of Traumatic Stress, 8,* 317–336.

Burstow, B. (2003). Towards a radical understanding of trauma and trauma work. *Violence Against Women, 9* (11), 1293–1317.

Carter, R. (2003). Sane responses: Exploring positive ways of working with mental health and domestic violence. Seminar Report. March, 2003. London: Greater London Domestic Violence Project.

Cascardi, M., O'Leary, K.D., & Schlee, K. (1999). Co-occurrence and correlates of posttraumatic stress disorder and major depression in physically abused women. *Journal of Family Violence, 14,* 227–249.

Charles, N. (2000). Feminism, the state and social policy. Basingstoke: Macmillan.

Chesler, P. (1972). Women and madness. New York: Doubleday Books.

Coker, A., Smith, P., Thompson, M., McKeown, R., Bethea, L., & Davis, K. (2002). Social support protects against the negative effects of partner violence on mental health. *Journal of Women's Health and Gender-Based Medicine, 11* (5), 465–476.

Davies, J. with Lyon, E., & Monti-Catania, D. (1998). Safety planning with battered women. London: Sage.

Davidson, J., Hughes, D., Blazer, D., & George, L. (1991). Post-traumatic stress disorder in the community: An epidemiological study. *Psychological Medicine, 21,* 713–721.

Department of Health. (2002). Women's mental health: Into the mainstream. London: Stationary Office. www.dh.gov.uk/mentalhealth

Department of Health. (1999). National service framework on mental health. London: Department of Health.

Dewees, M., Pulliam, R., & Roche, S. (2004). The view from the bridge: Advocacy and clinical practice. Fourth International Conference on Social Work in Health and Mental Health, Quebec, May 2004.

Flannery, K., Irwin, J., & Lopes, A. (2000). Connection and cultural difference: Women, groupwork and surviving domestic violence. *Women Against Violence, 9,* 14–21.

Fraser, N. (1989). Unruly practices: power, discourse and gender in contemporary social theory. Cambridge: Polity Press.

Gleason, W. (1993). Mental disorders in battered women: An empirical study. *Violence and Victims, 8,* 53–68.

Golding, J. (1999). Intimate partner violence as a risk factor for mental disorders: A meta analysis. *Journal of Family Violence, 14,* 99–132.

Hager, D. (2004). An investigation into the relationship between domestic violence and mental illness. Seminar paper. School of Health and Social Studies, University of Warwick, May 2004.

Hague, G., Mullender, A. & Aris, R. (2003). Is anyone listening? Accountability and women survivors of domestic violence. London: Routledge.

Hague, G., Malos, E., & Dear, W. (1996). Multi-agency work and domestic violence. Bristol: Policy Press.

Herbert, C., & Wetmore, A. (1999). Overcoming Traumatic Stress. London: Constable and Robinson.

Herman, J. (1992). Trauma and Recovery. New York: Basic Books.

Humphreys, C., & Harrison, C. (2003). Focusing on safety: Domestic violence and the role of child contact centres. *Child and Family Law Quarterly, 15* (3) 237–253.

Humphreys, C., & Thiara, R. (2003). Domestic violence and mental health: 'I call it symptoms of abuse'. *British Journal of Social Work, 33* (2), 209–226.

Humphreys, C., & Thiara, R. (2002). Routes to safety: Protection issues facing abused women and children and the role of outreach services. Bristol: Women's Aid Publications.

Johnson, M., & Ferraro, K. (2000). Research on domestic violence in the 1990s: Making distinctions. *Journal of Marriage and the Family, 4*, 948–963.

Jones, L., Highes, M., & Unterstaller, U. (2001). Post-traumatic stress disorder in victims of domestic violence: A review of the research. *Trauma, Violence and Abuse, 2* (2), 99–119.

Kemp, A., Green, B., Hovanitz, C., & Rawlings, E. (1995). Incidence and correlates of post-traumatic stress disorder in battered women: Shelter and community samples. *Journal of Interpersonal Violence, 10*, 43–55.

Laing, L. (2001). Working with women: Exploring individual and group work approaches. Issue Paper 4. Domestic Violence Clearinghouse. Sydney: University of New South Wales. www.austdvclearinghouse.unsw.edu.au

Lindy, J. (1996). Psychoanalytic psychotherapy of post-traumatic stress disorder: The nature of the relationship. In B. van der Kolk, A. McFarlane & L. Weisaeth (eds.), Traumatic stress: The effects of overwhelming experience on mind, body and society. (pp. 525–536). New York: Guilford Press.

Marmar, C., Weiss, D., & Pynoos, R. (1995). Dynamic psychotherapy of post-traumatic stress disorder. In M. Friedman, D. Charney & A. Deutch (eds.), Neurobiological and clinical consequences of stress: From normal adaptation to post traumatic stress disorder. (pp. 495–506). Philadelphia: Lippincott-Raven.

Marx, G., & McAdam, D. (1994). Collective behavior and social movements. Englewood Cliffs, NJ: Prentice-Hall.

Melucci, A. (1989.) Nomads of the present social movements and individual needs in contemporary society. Hutchinson: Radius.

Mitchell, J. (1983). When disaster strikes . . . . . The critical incident stress debriefing process. *Journal of Personality and Social Psychology, 50*, 1226–1234.

Merrill, J., & Owens, J. (1986). Ethnic differences in self-poisoning: A comparison of Asian and white groups. *British Journal of Psychiatry, 148*, 708–712.

Saunders, D. (1994). Post-traumatic stress symptom profiles of battered women: A comparison of survivors in two settings. *Violence and Victims, 9*, 31–44.

Palley, M. Medicalization versus de-medicalization of women's health. Fourth International Conference on Social Work in Health and Mental Health, Quebec, May 2004.

Resick, P. (2001). Stress and Trauma. Hove: Psychology Press.

Resick, P., & Jordan, C. (1988). Group stress inoculation training for victims of sexual assault: A therapist's manual. In P. Keller & S. Heyman (eds.), Innovations in clinical practice: A source book. Sarasota: Professional Resource Exchange.

Shapiro, F. (1989). Eye movement desensitization: A new treatment for post traumatic stress disorder. *Journal of Behaviour Therapy and Experimental Psychiatry, 20*, 211–217.

Shapiro, F. (1995). Eye movement desensitization and reprocessing: Basic principles, protocols and procedures. New York: Guilford.

Soni-Raleigh, V. (1996). Suicide patterns and trends in people of Indian Subcontinent and Carribbean origin in England and Wales. *Ethnicity and Health, 1*, 55–63.

Stanley, N., & Penhale, B. (1999). The mental health problems of mothers experiencing the child protection system: Identifying needs and appropriate responses. *Child Abuse Review, 8*, 34–45.

Stark, E., & Flitcraft, A. (1996). Women at risk: Domestic violence and women's health. London: Sage.

Stark, E., & Flitcraft, A. (1995). Killing the best within: Women battering and female suicidality. *International Journal of Health Services, 25*, 43–64.

Taft, A. (2003). Promoting women's mental health: The challenges of intimate/domestic violence against women. Issue Paper 8. New South Wales: Domestic Violence Clearinghouse. www.austdvclearinghouse.unsw.edu.au

Tarrier, N., Sommerfield, C., & Pilgrim, H. (1999). Relatives' expressed emotion (EE) and PTSD treatment outcome. *Psychological Medicine, 29*, 801–811.

Thompson, N. (2002). Social movements, social justice and social work. *British Journal of Social Work, 32*, 711–722.

Wilson, A. & Beresford, P. (2000) Anti-Oppressive Practice: Emancipation or Appropriation? *British Journal of Social Work, 30*, 553–73.

Yazdani, A. (1998). Young Asian women and self-harm: Mental health needs assessment of young Asian women in Newham. Newham Innercity Multifund and Newham Asian Women's Project.

Violence in the Lives of Lesbian Women: Implications for Mental Health

Batya Hyman, PhD

The mental health of lesbian women is shaped by the unique intersection of violence across the lifespan with the trauma of living in a heterosexist society. I argue that living within the heterosexist culture of the United States constitutes a form of trauma which is rarely considered when examining the mental health of lesbian women. Heterosexism is manifested at both individual and cultural levels. I discuss how the traumatic context created by heterosexism fosters the development of internalized homophobia and shapes the mental health of lesbian women. We must recognize that lesbians are not a homogenous group; there are significant within-group differences based on such factors as ethnicity, socioeconomic status, and age. These differences result in interlocking oppressions that influence mental health.

Lesbians experience violence across their lifespan. I discuss the mental health implications of the victimization of lesbian adolescents within their homes, schools, and communities. I then examine lesbian women's experiences, reported retrospectively, of childhood physical and sexual abuse perpetrated by family members and others. The experiences of lesbian and heterosexual women are compared and the impact on mental health is considered. The studies discussed in this paper were reported in social work, psychology, and medical journals prior to November 2004. Studies regarding violence, the lives of lesbian women across the lifespan, and mental health outcomes among lesbians are included. Studies that focused on violence within lesbian relationships or substance abuse among lesbian women were excluded.

HETEROSEXISM, INTERNALIZED HOMOPHOBIA, AND MENTAL HEALTH

Heterosexism has been defined as the ideological system that denies, denigrates, and stigmatizes any nonheterosexual identity, form of behavior, relationship, or community (Herek, 1990). Heterosexism may be described as heterosexuals' prejudices against lesbian women and gay men as well as the behaviors predicated on these prejudices (Herek, 1996).

"Cultural heterosexism, like institutional racism and sexism, pervades societal customs and institutions. It operates through a dual process of invisibility and attack." (Herek, 1996, p. 102) When people are identified as gay, they are subject to stigmatization and victimization by society. Examples of cultural heterosexism in the United States include the lack of legal protections for gays in the workplace, housing, and services; the military's "Don't Ask, Don't Tell" policy, which results in the dishonorable discharge of thousands of service people every year; and the failure to recognize lesbian and gay committed relationships.

INTERNALIZED HOMOPHOBIA AND MENTAL HEALTH OUTCOMES

From the time American children are very young, they are socialized with the anti-homosexual biases that are sanctioned by our culture (Gonsiorek, 1993). Children internalize these idealized values learned from their society and culture. When these idealized values do not match their experience of coming out, internal conflict can ensue (Pearlin, 1993). They realize that society disapproves of them. Lesbians incorporate these negative feelings into their self-image, which results in internalized homophobia (personal homonegativity). Internalized homophobia is defined as a set of negative attitudes and affects toward homosexual features in oneself. (Shidlo, 1994) Internalized homophobia can range from self doubt to overt self-hatred (Gonsiorek, 1993). Internalized homophobia can make lesbians feel that "the very center of their being is sick and disgusting" (Bobbe, 2002, p. 218).

Shidlo found that internalized homophobia explained a significant portion of "overall psychological distress, depression, somatic symptoms, self-esteem, and distrust" (1994, p. 198). However, in the course of coming out, most lesbian women successfully navigate the threats to psychological well-being posed by heterosexism. They cope with the need "to reclaim disowned or devalued parts of themselves, developing an identity into which their sexuality is well integrated" (Herek, 1996, p. 107).

MINORITY STRESS AS A CONSEQUENCE
OF HETEROSEXISM

Heterosexism is not experienced in the same way by all lesbians. Many lesbian women must integrate multiple identities. Greene (2000b) states that the African American community is perceived as homophobic by many of its lesbian members. She suggests that African Americans "may regard any sexual behavior outside of dominant cultural norms as reflecting negatively on African Americans as a group" (Greene, 2000b, p. 245). African Americans view gays as affluent, white, and endowed with both skin color and class privilege. Therefore many African Americans don't see how gays are oppressed. "Being gay is a chosen identity and inconvenience where being black is true hardship" (Greene, 2000a, p. 20). People of color feel that a comparison of heterosexism and racism as oppressions trivializes the history of racial oppression (Greene 2000a). Given this, lesbians of color are less likely to be out. They are, therefore, less visible to white lesbian women. Additionally, lesbians of color may not take for granted that they will be welcomed into the white lesbian community without continuing confrontations with racism.

In healthy African American families, children learn to view themselves positively because of loved and trusted family members' positive response to them as African Americans. This process affirms and reinforces for children the most important aspects of membership in their ethnic group (Greene, 2000b). African Americans and other families of color teach their children how to negotiate manifestations of racism. However, these families may be unable to teach them about how to negotiate homophobia. Lesbians and gay men must go outside of their families to develop an affirmative identity.

Unlike most other minority groups, lesbians are often not recognized as a legitimate minority group deserving of protections against discrimination. Lesbian stress is a form of minority stress. The stress that results from stigmatization often precipitates adverse life events over which the individual has no control (DiPlacido, 1998).

Mays and Cochran (2001) found a robust association between gay persons' experiences of lifetime and day-to-day discrimination and indicators of psychiatric morbidity. They suggest that extensive and destructive experiences of discrimination lie at the root of the somewhat greater prevalence of psychiatric morbidity among lesbians and gay men found in recent studies (Cochran & Mays, 1994; Fergussion, Horwood, & Beautrais, 1999).

MENTAL HEALTH IMPLICATIONS OF THE VICTIMIZATION OF YOUTHS

In this section we discuss aspects of the coming-out experience that are shaped by heterosexism, stigmatization, and internalized homophobia. Studies of these concerns sample either males alone or males and females. We will focus on reports of the experiences of lesbian youth who generally represent one third of study samples. The process of coming out often leads to amplified vulnerability to victimization within families and school settings.

COMING OUT AND HETEROSEXISM

The biological, psychological, and social changes related to puberty are stressful for many teenagers, but lesbian and gay youths face even more difficult challenges. By age 12, children have learned that heterosexuality is natural and that lesbianism is shameful. Youths are attacked with epithets like "you're so gay" or "you're a fag." According to an American Association of University Women report, being called "gay" by others was deemed the most upsetting form of sexual harassment in schools (AAUW, 1993). D'Augelli (1998) argues that youths with homoerotic feelings have experienced a "developmental opportunity loss"; that is, they are unable to positively resolve the developmental dilemma of puberty with an age-appropriate expression and exploration of homoerotic social and sexual relationships. They have also experienced "self-doubt induced by cultural heterosexism." "Self-acknowledgment of homoerotic feelings, itself the end point of a complex developmental process, instigates other processes of identity consolidation that are fundamentally social" (D'Augelli, 1998, p. 191).

The internalization of a devalued identity can erode coping efforts. Savin-Williams (1994) found three major problem areas. Lesbian youths have school problems because of harassment from other students, leading to excessive absences, poor academic performance, and dropping out. Lesbian youths may run away from home, and some wind up homeless. Lesbian youths abuse alcohol, drugs, and other substances to cope with daily stressors and with facing the future as a member of a stigmatized group. We do not have reliable empirical evidence regarding the adult consequences of living one's adolescence and early adulthood in self-doubt, fear, and alienation from self.

VICTIMIZATION IN FAMILIES

Pilkington and D'Augelli (1995) found that more than one third of their lesbian, gay, bisexual (LGB) sample of 194 youth between the ages of 15 and 21 had been verbally abused by a family member and 10% were physically assaulted by a family member because of their sexual orientation. Of those youths who were still living at home, one third of the lesbian youths who had disclosed their sexual orientation said that their mothers were verbally abusive; fathers were reported to be verbally abusive by 20 of the disclosed youths. Disclosed lesbian youths living at home were physically attacked by their parents—10% by mothers and 5% by fathers—more often than were the disclosed male youths—3% by mothers and 2% by fathers. Many reported fear of verbal or physical abuse at home.

VICTIMIZATION IN SCHOOL

Garofalo and colleagues (1998) used a representative sample of Massachusetts high school students to compare lesbian, gay, and bisexual identified youths with heterosexual students. One quarter of the LGB youths said they had missed school in the last month because of fear, compared to 5% of the non-LGB youths. One third of the LGB youths said they had been threatened with a weapon at school, compared with 7% of the other youths. Thirty-eight percent of the LGB youths were involved in fights at school, in contrast to 14% of the other students. And half of the LGB youths reported property damage at school compared with 29% of the other youths.

D'Augelli, Pilkington, and Hershberger (2002) studied 350 youths gathered from social and recreational groups for LGB youths located in the United States and Canada. The average age was 19 years old; only 7% were 14 to 17 years old. Forty-four percent of the sample were lesbian youths. The lesbian youths reported becoming first aware of their same-sex attraction at age 11 and self-labeled as lesbian at age 16. Current high school students were more open about their sexual orientation than college students were during their high school years. Students in high school reported higher overall victimization and verbal victimization compared to that experienced in high school by college students. Seven percent of the lesbian youths reported being assaulted because of their sexual orientation.

VICTIMIZATION AND THE MENTAL HEALTH
STATUS OF YOUTHS

D'Augelli, Pilkington, and Hershberger (2002) sampled 350 high school and college age youths. On the Personal Homonegativity Scale, participants had low overall negative views of their own sexual orientation. Ninety-four percent of the lesbian youths reported being glad to be lesbian. However, the researchers found that 25% of lesbians said they had sometimes or often thought of suicide. About half (48%) said their suicidal thinking was related to their sexual orientation. Over one third acknowledged a past suicide attempt. The earlier that youths were aware of their same-sex feelings, self identified as LGB, and disclosed their sexual orientation to others for the first time, the more they were victimized in high school. The overall number of years they had been out was also related significantly to increased victimization. In addition, the more open youths were about their sexual orientation in high school, the more they were victimized. Total victimization was related positively to mental health symptoms on the Brief Symptom Inventory and the Trauma Symptom Checklist.

Hershberger and D'Augelli (1995), employing an earlier sample of youths from recreation and social clubs across North America, found that positive adjustment in lesbian youths was associated with self-acceptance of their sexual orientation. A general sense of personal worth, coupled with a positive view of their sexual orientation, appeared to be critical for the youths' mental health. Even for youths who were fortunate to have family support and self-esteem, there existed a strong residual effect of victimization on mental health.

In the National Lesbian Health Care Survey (Bradford, Ryan, Rothblum (1994), mental health problems were common among the 17- to 24-year-old group. Sixty-two percent had received counseling. They reported most often concerns with family problems, depression, problems in relationships, and anxiety.

There is a disproportionally high incidence of suicide attempts among lesbian youths. Lewinsohn, Rohde, and Seeley (1996) have noted that lifetime suicide attempt rates in studies of all high school students range from 6% to 10%. In the National Lesbian Health Care Survey (Hyman, 2000), one quarter of the young lesbians had made a suicide attempt. Herdt and Boxer (1993) found that 53% of the lesbian youths in a Chicago youth support group program had made a suicide attempt compared with 20% of the gay male youths. Hershberger, Pilkington, and

D'Augelli (1997) found that 42% of the 194 youths reported a past suicide attempt. Attempters were aware of their sexual attractions at an earlier age, were more open about their sexual orientation, had lower self-esteem, and showed more current symptoms. Those who attempted suicide were also more often victimized than were others. The strongest correlations with past suicide attempts were the loss of friends due to sexual orientation and low self-esteem.

Many lesbian youths cope with the consequences of victimization by themselves or with a close circle of friends. For some youths, attacks may lead to an unexpected disclosure of their sexual orientation. Some youths have families who are uncomfortable with their child's sexual orientation. For these families, the victimization may compound problems within the family (Boxer, Cook, & Herdt, 1991).

CHILDHOOD VICTIMIZATION AND MENTAL HEALTH

In this section, studies of the prevalence of child abuse in lesbian women are reviewed, and the consequences of child abuse in these women are examined. Each study faces methodological limitations that are presented. A significant limitation is the inability to recruit a sample that is representative of all lesbian women. Some studies discussed here employ large representative samples with small proportions of lesbian and gay respondents. Others employ community-based convenience samples. Importantly, studies of lesbian women are not able to tap into the well of lesbians who are not out or who are out to only a select few people in their lives.

PREVALENCE OF CHILD SEXUAL ABUSE IN LESBIANS

During the 1980s three studies examined the rates of child sexual abuse among lesbian women. Loulan (1987) studied 1,566 lesbians who were primarily white and middle class. Their ages ranged from 25 to 60 years. Thirty-eight percent of these women experienced sexual abuse prior to age 18. Diana Russell (1983) interviewed 930 women in San Francisco. She did not ask the sexual orientation of the women; however, one may assume that a significant portion of her sample was lesbian. Thirty-eight percent of the women in her study experienced sexual abuse prior to age 18. Bradford and Ryan (1988) conducted the National Lesbian Health

Care Survey. This diverse sample of 1,925 lesbians completed question-naires. Thirty-two percent of these lesbian women reported child sexual abuse. Nineteen percent reported sexual abuse by relatives. These three studies reported correlations between childhood victimization and adverse psychological consequences—such as depression, anxiety, sui-cide attempts, poor self-esteem, difficulty trusting others, alcohol and drug abuse—in the adult lesbian women (Klinger & Stein, 1996).

Recent research provides evidence of conflicting findings regarding the prevalence of child sexual abuse in lesbians when compared with heterosexual women. Some studies have found higher rates of child sexual abuse among lesbians (Hughes et al., 2000; Lechner et al., 1993; Roberts & Sorenson, 1999). Others have found rates similar to those of women in the general population (Bradford, Ryan, & Rothblum, 1994; Brannock & Chapman, 1990; Peters & Cantrell, 1991; Rankow, Cambre, & Cooper, 1998; Weingourt, 1998). Differences in prevalence rates among both lesbians and women in the general population are likely due to variations in study methods and definitions, specificity and number of questions, and sample characteristics.

THE CONSEQUENCES OF CHILD MALTREATMENT

Hughes, Johnson, and Wilsnack (2001) studied a sample of 63 lesbian and 57 heterosexual women. Only one third of the sample was European American, which differs significantly from the usual samples of lesbians who are white, middle class, and well educated. Lesbians were recruited through a variety of sources including ads in newspapers, as well as contacts within organizations and informal social networks and events. During the initial telephone contact the lesbians were asked if they knew a heterosexual woman of the same race who had a job or role similar to their own, who might be willing to be interviewed. This technique was only partly successful and one third of the heterosexual women were recruited in a manner similar to the lesbians. There were no significant differences between the lesbian and heterosexual women on demographic measures.

This research team administered the Health and Life Experiences of Women instrument to the fourth wave of subjects. This interview instrument was developed to gather data about the alcohol use and abuse behaviors of women, including those factors known to predict substance use such as child sexual abuse. Sexual orientation questions were added to the instrument in 1996 and it is that data that the team reports.

In this study by Hughes and colleagues (2001), more lesbian (68%) than heterosexual (47%) women reported sexually abusive behavior occurring prior to age 18. In addition, more lesbian (37%) than heterosexual (19%) women reported they perceived themselves as having been sexually abused as a child. There was a trend, though not significant, toward a greater number of lesbians reporting intrafamilial abuse.

Lesbians are assumed to be at heightened risk for alcohol abuse as a consequence of cultural and environmental factors associated with being stigmatized and marginalized (Hughes et al., 2001). Thirteen percent of the heterosexual women were lifetime abstainers; none of the lesbians were. Four percent of the heterosexual women were 12-month abstainers; 25% of the lesbians were. More lesbian (18%) than heterosexual (2%) women reported they were in recovery. Forty-seven percent of the lesbians and 16% of the heterosexual women reported that they have wondered at some point in the past whether they might have a drinking problem. The researchers note that the majority of lesbians in the study did not drink excessively or experience alcohol-related problems.

Child sexual abuse was associated with lifetime alcohol abuse, to a similar and significant degree, in both the lesbian and heterosexual women, a finding that supports results from research with women in the general population (Wilsnack, Vogeltanz, Klassen, & Harris, 1997). The rate of child sexual abuse among the lesbians in this study (25%) was similar to rates reported for lesbians in the National Lesbian Health Care Survey (32%) (Bradford & Ryan, 1988) and in the Boston Health Project (21%) (Roberts & Sorensen, 1999).

Hyman (2000) investigated the relation between a lesbian woman's experience of childhood sexual victimization and her economic welfare as an adult. She analyzed data from the National Lesbian Health Care Survey (Bradford & Ryan, 1988), which gathered information from 1925 participants about experiences of childhood victimization, adult health status, mental health status, and economic welfare. The child sexual abuse survivors reported a greater number of health and mental health problems than the other lesbian women. They were receiving treatment for a larger number of health problems. They reported higher rates of depression, anxiety, and attempted suicide. Survivors of intrafamilial abuse were more likely to have a history of mental health hospitalization.

Additionally, the survivors did not attain as much education as the others. They were less likely to work, less likely to work full-time, and less likely to choose high-status occupations. The child sexual abuse survivors also reported lower earnings. Estimation of the simultaneous equation model revealed that the experience of child sexual abuse adversely affected the health, mental health, educational attainment, and annual earnings of the survivors.

By shifting the emphasis from isolated aspects of a woman's life, such as her psychological functioning, to an integrated examination of the major spheres of her life, this model moves away from a simple cataloguing of consequences and toward a richer appreciation of how child sexual abuse affects several dimensions of the adult's functioning.

Hall (1999) conducted qualitative interviews with eight lesbian survivors of child sexual abuse. She found that the lesbian women described their identities as survivor and lesbian as a double secret to be kept. These women also reported a lack of sexual spontaneity with their partners. Three of the women reported being sexually assaulted by another woman during adulthood.

Tomeo, Templer, Anderson, and Kotler (2001) compared the incidence of childhood sexual abuse in 942 heterosexual and homosexual men and women. Four hundred sixty heterosexual female students and 153 lesbians participated. Nearly all of the lesbians were recruited through gay pride festivals. On average, the women were 30 years old and had 15 years of schooling. Clearly this is not a representative sample.

Respondents were asked "did you ever have sexual contact with a . . ." Of course, sexual contact and sexual abuse are not necessarily the same. Since the female victims in this study had a mean age of 13 at the time of sexual contact and 68% of them were at least 12 years old, we are dealing with adolescent sexual contact. By definition, the perpetrators were at least 16 years old and five years older than the victims. Using these parameters, one quarter of the heterosexual women reported being sexually abused as a child; 24.3% by a man and 1.1% by a woman. Forty-two percent of the lesbian women reported molestation, 29% by men and 22% by women.

Tjaden, Thoennes, and Allison (1999) studied violence against children and adults in a nationally representative sample of same-sex and opposite-sex cohabitants, the National Violence Against Women Survey of November 1995 through May 1996. Participants were not asked their sexual orientation, but were instead asked to identify whether they lived with someone of the same or opposite sex as well as information about their past live-in relationships. A total of 8,000 women and 8,000 men were interviewed using a computer-assisted telephone interviewing system. One percent of all women surveyed (N = 79) reported they had lived with a same-sex partner "as a couple" at some time in their lives. Several screening questions were asked regarding sexual victimization and a modified form of the Conflict Tactics Scale was used.

Differences between the opposite-sex cohabiting and same-sex cohabiting female samples were noted. Same-sex cohabiting women tended to be younger than opposite-sex cohabiting women, a factor that may predispose them to higher rates of abuse. Same-sex cohabiting women also tended to have more education, more full time employment, and somewhat higher incomes, factors that are inversely association with victimization.

The same-sex cohabiting women were nearly twice as likely as opposite-sex cohabiting women to report sexual assault as a minor (16.5% versus 8.7%). Same-sex cohabiting women were significantly more likely to report being physically assaulted as a child by an adult caretaker (59.5% versus 35.7%). Further, the physical abuse reported by same-sex cohabitants was more severe. Over half (53.2%) of the same-sex cohabiting women reported being physically assaulted as an adult compared to only 29.7% of the opposite-sex cohabiting women. Additional findings regarding domestic violence were presented.

Corliss, Cochran, and Mays (2002) investigated the prevalence and nature of childhood maltreatment experiences among lesbian, gay, and heterosexual adults. The self-administered questionnaire data was collected as part of the 1996 National Survey of Midlife Development in the United States. Parental maltreatment behaviors were adapted from 3 subscales of the Conflict Tactics Scale. Respondents were asked to self-identify as heterosexual (n = 2844), homosexual (n = 41), or bisexual (n = 32). Lesbian and bisexual women, 2.2% of the sample (n = 37), were grouped together for the purpose of analysis. The lesbian/bi women differed from the heterosexual women on two important demographic factors, age, and annual income. The lesbian/bi women were younger and earned more than the heterosexual women.

The rate of abuse by either parent was 43.6% for the lesbian/bi women and 30.9% for the heterosexual women. The lesbian and bisexual women reported more physical maltreatment by their mothers (32.8% versus 23.7%). The rate of major physical maltreatment by mothers was greater among the lesbian/bi women as well (22.8% versus 6.9%). The lesbian/bi women reported more physical maltreatment by their fathers (27.2% versus 18.6%). Again the rate of major physical abuse by fathers was greater among the lesbian/bi women (15.1% versus 5.8%). The prevalence of major physical maltreatment by either parent was dramatically higher among the lesbian/bi group (33.6% versus 10.3%). Clearly, lesbian and bisexual women are more likely than heterosexual women to report childhood histories of parental maltreatment. These findings are supported by other research (Faulkner & Cranston, 1998; Garofalo et al., 1998; Saewye et al., 1998).

MENTAL HEALTH STATUS OF LESBIANS

We now take up three studies that examine the factors that contribute to a lesbian woman's mental health status.

Hughes, Haas, Razzano, Cassidy, and Matthews (2000) compare the mental health functioning of lesbian and heterosexual women. The survey questionnaire was developed by an interdisciplinary team and piloted in Chicago. Nearly all data gathered were based on closed-ended questions. In order to collect a diverse sample of women, the research team asked lesbians who completed the survey to give a second copy to a heterosexual woman with a role as similar as possible to the lesbian's own. In one city the women were given a small incentive for recruiting heterosexual work/role mates.

Rather than rely on one difinition of sexual orientation or ask the women to self-identify, two questions were included in the survey instrument dealing with sexual attraction, sexual behavior, and sexual identity. This allowed the research team to define sexual orientation "more systematically" (Hughes et al., 2000). Based on this schema, 550 women were categorized as lesbian, 279 as heterosexual, and 33 as bisexual. The mean age of the sample was 42.5 years old. Seventy-six percent of the lesbians and 72% of the heterosexual women were European American, and 12% of the lesbians and 14% of the heterosexual women were African American. The same proportions of lesbian and heterosexual women (52%) reported living with a partner or spouse. Sixty-six percent of the lesbian women reported being in a committed relationship.

Both the lesbian and heterosexual women reported moderate levels of stress. Lesbians rated job, money, and overall responsibilities as the highest sources of stress. The only significant differences in the sources of stress between the two groups of women was that the heterosexual women rated children as the biggest source of stress and the lesbian women rated sexual identity the highest.

The two groups of women were equally likely to report they had "ever been a victim of non-sexual physical violence" (45% and 41%). A family member was the most commonly reported perpetrator, especially a sex partner. The majority of these women reported the physical violence occurred more than five years ago.

Forty-one percent of lesbian women and 24% of the heterosexual women reported an experience of child sexual abuse before age 15 (p < .001).

Fifty-six percent of lesbian women and 49% of heterosexual women reported depression as a reason for seeking therapy. Twenty-six percent of lesbian women and 20% of heterosexual women reported taking medication for a mental health problem. Mast had taken antidepressants. Fifty-eight percent of the lesbian and 52% of the heterosexual women reported at least one of these two indicators of past depression. There were significant differences between the lesbian (51%) and heterosexual women (38%) in the rates of suicidal ideation. Further, significantly more lesbians (22%) than heterosexuals (13%) reported prior suicide attempts.

Lesbians were significantly more likely to have received therapy or counseling (78% and 56%). The majority of both lesbian and heterosexual women who had sought therapy had done so during their 20s or 30s. In both groups, the most common reason for seeking therapy was for problems with a spouse or partner. Lesbians also reported problems with their sexual identity, suicidal ideation, sexual abuse, and problems related to substance use. Almost all of the lesbians and 70% of the heterosexual women reported having a female therapist as important. The same proportions of lesbian and heterosexual women (52%) reported living with a partner or spouse. Sixty-six percent of the lesbian women reported being in a committed relationship.

Lesbians were more likely than heterosexuals to report abstinence from alcohol during the prior 12 months (24% and 17%). This supports findings from other studies (Heffernan, 1998; Saulnier & Miller, 1997). Seventy-three percent of the lesbian and 82% of the heterosexual women reported light to moderate drinking levels at the time of the study. The two groups were similar in their reports of at least one indicator of problem drinking during the past year. Significantly, 14% of the lesbians and 6% of heterosexuals indicated they sought help for alcohol or drug problems in the past.

The study authors speculate that the lesbians' high rates of seeking mental health services may serve as a buffer against stress and the resulting depression.

The experience of coming out may have influenced several of the study findings. The lesbian women reported suicide attempts during the ages of 15–19, during the years they may have self-identified as lesbian. Also, younger lesbian women were at highest risk for alcohol problems. Perhaps age also influenced perceptions of stress. Would contemporary younger lesbian women who are maturing during the recent period of greater visibility of lesbians still rate sexual identity as the highest source of stress?

Matthews, Hughes, Johnson, Razzano, and Cassidy (2002) investigated the predictors of depression in a community sample of lesbian and heterosexual women. They employed data from the Hughes et al., (2000) study reviewed above to examine whether sexual orientation is a predictor of depressive symptoms such as a history of seeking therapy, treatment for depression, a history of suicidal ideation, and a history of suicide attempts. They tested several assumed predictors of depression including experiences of physical violence and child sexual abuse, perceived level of stress, global stress, lack of social support, and coping strategies.

The majority of the women were white, were married or involved in a committed relationship, had more than a high school education, and were employed full time for pay. The median household income for both lesbians and heterosexual women was $36,000 to $50,999.

The lesbian and heterosexual women were equally likely to report being a victim of nonsexual physical violence. Lesbian women were more likely than heterosexual women to report experiences of child sexual abuse (30% and 16%).

Overall mean scores on the global stress index were in the lower range and did not differ according to sexual orientation. The lesbian and heterosexual women all reported moderate to extreme levels of perceived stress. The only significant differences in sources of stress for the lesbian and heterosexual women involved children and sexual identity. The heterosexual women rated children as moderately or extremely stressful. The lesbian women rated sexual identity as moderately or extremely stressful.

More heterosexual women (6%) than lesbians (3%) reported an absence of social support. The use of positive coping strategies was low among both groups of women. Lesbians were significantly more likely to report never using talking as a coping strategy (46% versus 37%). Fewer lesbians (19%) than heterosexual women (25%) reported doing something fun when they were stressed or using exercise as a coping strategy (36% vs. 43%). Equally few lesbian and heterosexual women reported confronting situations directly.

The logistic regression analyses successfully identified factors which contributed to each of the four depression variables: whether the woman ever sought counseling, whether the woman participated in counseling for depression, a history of suicidal ideation, and a history of suicide attempts. We are particularly interested in three of the explanatory factors: lesbian sexual orientation, high stress levels, and a history of child physical or sexual abuse. All three of these factors predicted each of the four depression variables with one exception. High stress levels did not predict a history of suicide attempts.

Lesbian sexual orientation was a significant predictor of all four depression measures. The researchers speculate that other factors not included in their models may in part account for the association between sexual orientation and depressive distress. "For example, self-esteem, internalized homophobia, level of social support, and religious attitudes and beliefs may be important variables that moderate or mediate the relationship between sexual orientation and depressive distress" (Matthews et al., 2002, p. 1137). Additionally they state that it is not clear whether the sexual orientation's power is conferred through the long-term chronic stress associated with membership in a stigmatized minority group or through more time-limited stressful life circumstances such as coming out.

Razzano, Matthews, and Hughes (2002) compare the use of mental health services by lesbian and heterosexual women. They employed data from the Wilsnack et al., 1997 study described above. The sample consisted of 63 lesbians and 57 matched heterosexual women. The average age of the women was 40 years old. Only 37% of the sample was European American. Twenty eight percent were African American, 25% were Latina, 7% were Asian, and 3% were American Indian. Fifty-seven percent were married or in a committed relationship. Fifty-eight percent were working full-time for pay.

There were no significant differences between lesbian and heterosexual women on variables such as anxiety, sexual problems, insomnia, problems with alcohol/drugs, behavioral problems of children, or relationship concerns.

Descriptive data analyses indicated significant differences in the proportion of lesbians (70%) compared to heterosexual women (44%) who reported any use of mental health services during the prior 5 years as well as any use of substance-related services in the past 5 years (23% vs. 4%). Contrary to other studies, no significant differences were found between lesbian and heterosexual women regarding their ability to obtain mental health services, past history of child sexual experience, past history of physical abuse, or current use of antidepressant use. Lesbians were significantly more likely than heterosexual women to seek services for reasons related to depression and sexual orientation.

CONCLUSION

Lesbian women are thought to be at greater risk for mental health problems than are heterosexual women (Bradford, Ryan, & Rothblum, 1994; Cochran & Mays, 1994; Hyman, 2000; Rothblum, 1994; Trippet, 1994). This is borne out by the studies reviewed here. Lesbians are believed to be affected by additional, unique risk factors, including the "coming out" process, level of disclosure of sexual orientation, discrimination experiences, and chronic stress associated with being a member of a stigmatized minority group (Ayala & Coleman, 2000; Octjen & Rothblum, 2000; Rothblum, 1990; Tait, 1997). Several of the studies reviewed here report similar findings. We need to learn more about the impact of living with multiple forms of minority stress.

Some researchers have found higher rates of childhood maltreatment among lesbians when compared with heterosexual women. Why might lesbian women be more likely to have a history of childhood physical and sexual abuse? Hughes, et al. (2001) speculate that lesbian women may be more likely to acknowledge and disclose both their sexual identity and other stigmatized statuses or experiences. Research shows that lesbian women are more likely to engage in therapy which may increase their willingness to be open.

How do lesbian women come to terms with their experiences of childhood victimization? How does this childhood experience shape one's coming out process and possibility of internalizing homophobia? Matthews et al. (2002) point out that past traumatic experiences, such as physical or sexual abuse, may add to the vulnerability of young lesbians who may be struggling with issues related to coming out and may increase the risk of suicide.

We need to expand our research with lesbian youth. More lesbian youth will, in the future, disclose their sexual orientation to others, and at earlier ages. As youths self-label earlier they will experience greater vulnerability in unfriendly school settings. The increased visibility of lesbian and gay people in our society may open a new vista for lesbian youth. It may also stimulate a backlash. Will this endanger lesbian youths? We must think about the supports lesbian youths will need available to them in the coming years. Studies should be undertaken with today's youth and tomorrow's youth because our environment is changing so quickly.

The studies reviewed here suffer from methodological limitations. As discussed earlier, we cannot collect a representative sample of lesbian women. In addition, the studies employ different definitions of lesbian, childhood maltreatment, stress, and mental health. Each study uses different measures of similar concepts. Many of these studies gather retrospective data regarding childhood victimization and adolescent experiences of violence and coming out. We must consider how experiences during the intervening years have colored memories. We do not know now how self-identifying as a lesbian affects the perception of past experiences.

According to all of the studies reviewed here, *most lesbian women exhibit mental well-being.* In the course of coming out, most lesbian women successfully navigate the threats to psychological well-being posed by heterosexism and internalized homophobia. They cope with the need "to reclaim disowned or devalued parts of themselves, developing an identity into which their sexuality is well integrated" (Herek, 1996, p. 107). DiPlacido (1998) comments that minority stress may lead to negative health outcomes among some members of sexual minorities, but we must remember that not all members of sexual minorities experience adverse physical and mental health consequences as a result of their minority status. Instead, many lesbian women demonstrate a kind of resilience found among many members of marginalized groups (Greene, 2000a). One characteristic of resilient people, including abuse survivors, is their capacity to evoke affirming reactions from others (Hyman & Williams, 2001). The lesbian and gay community provides some of this support.

Most Americans now believe that lesbian women and gay men deserve civil rights and protections. The United States and Canada are engaged in heated debates about same-sex marriage. How will such changes in the climate shape heterosexism, minority stress, the victimization of youths? And, how will these newly formed processes affect the mental health of lesbian youths, adults, and elders in the coming years? The increased visibility and political foothold of lesbian women and gay men provides an exciting new backdrop for new research.

REFERENCES

American Association of University Women. (1993). *Hostile hallways: The AAUW survey on sexual harassment in America's schools.* Washington, DC: Author.

American Medical Association Council on Scientific Affairs. (1996). Health care needs of gay men and lesbians in the United States: Council report. *Journal of the American Medical Association, 275*(17), 1354–1359.

Ayala, J., & Coleman, H. (2000). Predictors of depression among lesbian women. *Journal of Lesbian Studies, 4*(3), 71–86.

Bobbe, J. (2002). Treatment with lesbian alcoholics: Healing shame and internalized homophobia for ongoing sobriety. *Health and Social Work, 27*(3), 218–222.

Boxer, A. M., Cook, J. A., & Herdt, B. (1991). Double jeopardy: Identity transitions and parent-child relations among gay and lesbian youth. In K. Pillemer & K. McCartney (Eds.), *Parent-child relations throughout life* (pp. 59–92). Hillsdale, NJ: Lawrence Erlbaum.

Bradford, J., & Ryan, C. (1988). *National Lesbian Health Care Survey: Final Report.* Washington, D.C.: National Lesbian and Gay Health Foundation.

Bradford, J., Ryan, C., & Rothblum, E. D. (1994). National Lesbian Health Care Survey: Implications for mental health care. *Journal of Consulting and Clinical Psychology, 62*(2), 228–242.

Brannock, J. C., & Chapman, B. E. (1990). Negative sexual experiences with men among heterosexual women and lesbians. *Journal of Homosexuality, 19*, 195–210.

Cochran, S. D., & Mays, V. M. (1994). Depressive distress among homosexually active African American men and women. *American Journal of Psychiatry, 151*, 524–529.

Corliss, H. L., Cochran, S.D. & Mays, V.M. (2002). Reports of parental maltreatment during childhood in a United States population-based survey of homosexual, bisexual, and heterosexual adults. *Child Abuse & Neglect, 26*, 1165–1178.

D'Augelli, A. R. (1998). Developmental implications of victimization of lesbian, gay, and bisexual youths. In G. M. Herek (Ed.), *Stigma and sexual orientation: Understanding prejudice against lesbians, gay men, and bisexuals* (pp. 187–210). Thousand Oaks, CA: Sage Publications.

D'Augelli, A. R., Grossman, A. H., Hershberger, S. L., & O'Connell, T. S. (2001). Aspects of mental health among older lesbian, gay, and bisexual adults. *Aging and Mental Health, 5*(2), 149–158.

D'Augelli, A. R., Pilkington, N. W., & Hershberger, S. L. (2002). Incidence and mental health impact of sexual orientation victimization of lesbian, gay, and bisexual youths in high school. *School Psychology Quarterly, 17*(2), 148–167.

DiPlacido, J. (1998). Minority stress among lesbians, gay men, and bisexuals: A consequence of heterosexism, homophobia, and stigmatization. In G. M. Herek (Ed.), *Stigma and sexual orientation: Understanding prejudice against lesbians, gay men, and bisexuals* (pp. 138–159). Thousand Oaks, CA: Sage Publications.

Faulkner, A. H., & Cranston, K. (1998). Correlates of same-sex sexual behavior in a random sample of Massachusetts high school students. *American Journal of Public Health, 88*, 262–266.

Fergusson, D. M., Horwood, L. J., & Beautrais, A. L. (1999). Is sexual orientation related to mental health problems and suicidality in young people? *Archives of General Psychiatry, 56*, 876–880.

Garofalo, R., Wolf, R. C., Kessel, S., Palfrey, S. J., & DuRant, R. H. (1998). The association between health risk behaviors and sexual orientation among a school-based sample of adolescents. *Pediatrics, 101*, 895–902.

Gonsiorek, J. C. (1993). Threat, stress, and adjustment mental health and the workplace for gay and lesbian individuals. In L. Diamant (Ed.), *Homosexual issues in the workplace* (pp. 243–264). Washington, DC: Taylor and Francis.

Gonsiorek, J. C. (1993). Mental health issues of gay and lesbian adolescents. In L. D. Garnets & D. C. Kimmel (Eds.), *Psychological perspectives on lesbian and gay male experiences* (pp. 469–485). New York: Columbia University Press.

Greene, B. (2000). Beyond heterosexism and across the cultural divide: Developing an inclusive lesbian, gay, and bisexual psychology: A look to the future. In B. Greene & G. L. Croom (Eds.), *Education, research, and practice in lesbian, gay, bisexual, and transgendered psychology: A resource manual* (pp. 1–45). Thousand Oaks: Sage Publications.

Hall, J. (1999). An exploration of the sexual and relationship experiences of lesbian survivors of childhood sexual abuse. *Sexual and Marital Therapy, 14*(1), 61–70.

Heffernan, K. (1998). The nature and predictors of substance abuse among lesbians. *Addictive Behaviors, 23*(4), 517–528.

Herdt, G. H., & Boxer, A. M. (1993). *Children of Horizons: How gay and lesbian teens are leading a new way out of the closet.* Boston: Beacon Press.

Herek, G. M. (1990). The context of anti-gay violence: Notes on cultural and psychological heterosexism. *Journal of Interpersonal Violence, 5*, 316–333.

Herek, G. M. (1996). Heterosexism and homophobia. In R. P. Cabaj & T. S. Stein (Eds.), *Textbook of Homosexuality and Mental Health* (pp. 101–113). Washington, D.C.: American Psychiatric Press.

Hershberger, S. L., & D'Augelli, A. R. (1995). The impact of victimization on the mental health and suicidality of lesbian, gay, and bisexual youths. *Developmental Psychology, 31*(1), 65–74.

Hershberger, S. L., Pilkington, N. W., & D'Augelli, A. R. (1997). Predictors of suicide attempts among gay, lesbian, and bisexual youth. *Journal of Adolescent Research, 12*(4), 477–497.

Hughes, T. L., Haas, A. P., Razzano, L., Cassidy, R., & Matthews, A. (2000). Comparing lesbians' and heterosexual women's mental health: A multi-site survey. *Journal of Gay and Lesbian Social Services, 11*(1), 57–76.

Hughes, T. L., Johnson, T., & Wilsnack, S. C. (2001). Sexual assault and alcohol abuse: A comparison of lesbians and heterosexual women. *Journal of Substance Abuse, 13*, 515–532.

Hyman, B. (2000). The economic consequences of child sexual abuse for adult lesbian women. *Journal of Marriage and the Family, 62*, 199–211.

Hyman, B., & Williams, L. (2001). Resilience in adult female survivors of child sexual abuse. *Affilia: Journal of Women and Social Work.*

Klinger, R. L., & Stein, T. S. (1996). Impact of violence, childhood sexual abuse, and domestic violence and abuse on lesbians, bisexuals, and gay men. In R. P. Cabaj & T. S. Stein (Eds.), *Textbook of homosexuality and mental health* (pp. 801–818). Washington, DC: American Psychiatric Press.

Lechner, M. E., Vogel, M. E., Garcia-Shelton, L. M., Leichter, O. L., & Steibel, K. R. (1993). Self-reported medical problems of adult female survivors of childhood sexual abuse. *Journal of Family Practice, 36*, 633–638.

Lewinsohn, P. M., Rohde, P., & Seeley, J. R. (1996). Adolescent suicide ideation and attempts: Prevalence, risk factors, and clinical implications. *Clinical Psychology: Science and Practice, 3*, 25–46.

Loulan, J. (1987). *Lesbian passion*. San Francisco: Spinsters/Aunt Lute Books.

Matthews, A. K., Hughes, T. L., Johnson, T., Razzano, L. A., & Cassidy, R. (2002). Prediction of depressive distress in a community sample of women: The role of sexual orientation. *American Journal of Public Health, 92*(7), 1131–1139.

Mays, V. M., & Cochran, S. D. (2001). Mental health correlates of perceived discrimination among lesbian, gay, and bisexual adults in the United States. *American Journal of Public Health, 91*(11), 1869–1876.

Octjen, H., & Rothblum, E. D. (2000). When lesbians aren't gay: Factors affecting depression among lesbians. *Journal of Homosexuality*.

Pearlin, L. I. (1993). The social context of stress. In L. Goldberger & S. Breznitz (Eds.), *Handbook of stress: Theoretical and clinical aspects* (pp. 303–315). New York: Free Press.

Peters, D. K., & Cantrell, P. J. (1991). Factors distinguishing samples of lesbian and heterosexual women. *Journal of Homosexuality, 21*, 1–15.

Pilkington, N. W., & D'Augelli, A. R. (1995). Victimizations of lesbian, gay, and bisexual youth in community settings. *Journal of Community Psychology, 23*, 34–56.

Rankow, E. J., Cambre, K. M., & Cooper, K. (1998). Health care-seeking behavior of adult lesbian and bisexual survivors of childhood sexual abuse. *Journal of the Gay and Lesbian Medical Association, 2*(2), 69–76.

Razzano, L., Matthews, A. & Hughes, T. (2002). Utilization of mental health services: A comparison of lesbian and heterosexual women. *Journal of Gay & Lesbian Social Services, 14*(1), 51–66.

Roberts, S. J., & Sorensen, L. (1999). Prevalence of childhood sexual abuse and related sequelae in a lesbian population. *Journal of the Gay and Lesbian Medical Association, 3*(1), 11–19.

Rothblum, E. D. (1990). Depression among lesbians: An invisible and unresearched phenomenon. *Journal of Gay and Lesbian Psychotherapy, 1*(3), 67–87.

Rothblum, E. D. (1994). Lesbians and physical appearance: Which model applies? In B. Greene & G. M. Herek (Eds.), *Lesbian and gay psychology: Theory, research, and clinical applications* (Vol. 1, pp. 84–97). Thousand Oaks, CA: Sage Publications.

Russell, D. E. H. (1983). The incidence and prevalence of intrafamilial and extrafamilial sexual abuse of female children. *Child Abuse and Neglect, 7*, 133–146.

Saewyc, E. M., Bearinger, L., Heinz, P. A., Blum, R. W., & Resnick, M. D. (1998). Gender differences in health and risk behaviors among bisexual and homosexual adolescents. *Journal of Adolescent Health, 23*(3), 181–188.

Saulnier, C. F., & Miller, B. A. (1997). Drug and alcohol problems: Heterosexual compared to lesbian and bisexual women. *Canadian Journal of Human Sexuality*, 221–231.

Savin-Williams, R. C. (1994). Verbal and physical abuse as stressors in the lives of lesbian, gay male, and bisexual youths: Associations with school problems, running away, substance abuse, prostitution, and suicide. *Journal of Consulting and Clinical Psychology, 62*, 261–269.

Schulman, S. (1994). *My American history: Lesbian and gay life during the Reagan/Bush years*. New York: Routledge.

Shidlo, A. (1994). Internalized homophobia: Conceptual and empirical issues in measurement. In B. Greene & G. M. Herek (Eds.), *Lesbian and gay psychology: Theory, research, and clinical applications* (Vol. 1, pp. 176–205). Thousand Oaks, CA: Sage Publications.

Tait, D. (1997). Stress and social support networks among lesbian and heterosexual women: A comparison study. *Smith College Studies in Social Work, 67*(2), 213–224.

Tjaden, P., Thoennes, N., & Allison, C. J. (1999). Comparing violence over the life span in samples of same-sex and opposite-sex cohabitants. *Violence and Victims, 14*(4), 413–425.

Tomeo, M. E., Templer, D. I., Anderson, S., & Kotler, D. (2001). Comparative data of childhood and adolescence molestation in heterosexual and homosexual persons. *Archives of Sexual Behavior, 30*(5), 535–541.

Trippet, S. E. (1994). Lesbians' mental health concerns. *Health Care Women International, 15*, 317–323.

Weingourt, R. (1998). A comparison of heterosexual and homosexual long-term sexual relationships. *Archives of Psychiatric Nursing, 12*, 114–118.

Wilsnack, S. C., Vogeltanz, N. D., Klassen, A. D., & Harris, T. R. (1997). Childhood sexual abuse and women's substance abuse: National survey findings. *Journal of Studies on Alcohol, 58*, 264–271.

Reclaiming Stolen Identities: Resilience and Social Justice in Mid-Life

Carol Irizarry, PhD

"Immigration is accompanied by a deep sense of loss. One loses one's homeland, family, friends, culture and language which occupied not only one's everyday life, but more importantly, one's self-identity and the internal representations of one's objects."

(Mirsky, 1991, p. 618)

THE FORMER BRITISH CHILD MIGRANTS IN AUSTRALIA

Estimates vary on the number of British children sent to Australia as unaccompanied minors in the 20th century, but according to the Australian Department of Immigration and Multicultural Affairs that number is between 6,000 and 7,500 children (Senate Community Affairs Reference Committee, 2001, p. 69). Of this number about 3,000 to 3,500 were sent before World War II and 3,000 to 3,500 were sent after World War II. All of these children had been in care agencies in the United Kingdom and were transferred to Australia through a number of Acts passed in both countries.

In the Empire Settlement Act of 1922 the United Kingdom government initiated schemes with the Dominion Governments in the British Commonwealth countries which provided subsidized fares for children sent overseas by voluntary societies in Britain. The Act also made funds available to nongovernment organizations for child migration activities (Commonwealth of Australia, 2001).

Prior to World War II immigration schemes in Australia were handled by State Immigration Department in each of the five States but the Australian Commonwealth government contributed subsidy towards any child migrants. This contribution could go to any receiving agency selected by the state government (Commonwealth of Australia, 2001).

After World War II in 1946, the Empire Settlement Act was re-activated in Britain and two years later in 1948 the Child Act was passed, which gave the United Kingdom Secretary of State the legal power to approve emigration of children from voluntary care organizations to Australia and to allow local authorities to arrange their transport. Both the British and Australian governments entered into agreements with Australian receiving agencies.

In Australia the Immigration Guardianship of Children Act in 1946 was passed by the Commonwealth government which gave the Minister of Immigration legal guardianship of unaccompanied child migrants until they reached age 21. This authority was delegated to State Welfare authorities and the State governments delegated care and welfare of children to voluntary organizations, many of them church-based agencies. Sherington & Jeffery (1998) reported that 1,898 children were placed in church agencies in Australia, ranging in age from 5 to 15 years. They had come from various Catholic orphanages around England (Sherington & Jeffery, 1998).

Of these children about 62 went to the State of South Australia, 47 being placed in the Goodwood Orphanage in the capital city of Adelaide. This orphanage was run by the Sisters of Mercy, an order of the Roman Catholic Church. The women who are the Former British Child Migrants (FBCM) in this report arrived in Adelaide on the Ormandie boat in January of 1949.

INITIAL CONTACT WITH THE FORMER FORMER BRITISH CHILD MIGRANTS

The Flinders University of South Australia School of Social Work established a Loss and Grief Centre in partnership with Anglicare South Australia in 2000, with the university role focused on helping to identify, and developing services for, groups in the community with loss, grief, and trauma experiences who might not be receiving mainstream services. Various visits were made and pamphlets dispersed around the Adelaide social welfare agencies.

Early in 2001 a phone call was received at the Centre from a Former British Child Migrant who had been part of the Goodwood Orphanage contingent. This woman, now in her 60s, had been in the Adoption and Family Information Unit of the South Australian Department of Human Services seeking help and information on her background and had seen the pamphlet on the Loss and Grief Centre. She said on the phone that it seemed as if loss and grief were the feelings that she and many of her friends had lived with for many years. A meeting was arranged and within weeks a new group had been established at the centre for the Former British Child Migrants.

The women who attended the first meeting asked for a place to be their "home" for regular meetings—a place where their experiences would be acknowledged but not totally define who they were. They also asked that the interest we showed in them be sustained, stating that the Former British Child Migrants had recently received publicity that had given them a "flash in the pan of public media" but no lasting help with living with their past. The Loss and Grief Centre agreed to host the group and supply a part-time social worker. The group has continued to meet monthly since that time.

From the beginning of an encounter with these remarkable women the contradictions embedded in their lives were obvious. One could see such resilience in surviving the harshness of their childhoods but also the deeply embedded grief and anger at those experiences which had been largely ignored by society, and the resulting effects of trauma suffered at an early age. It was in juxtaposing and balancing these divergent themes that the work was concentrated—that is, the interactive effects of resilience, trauma, loss, grief, and social justice.

THEIR RESILIENCE

"Nowadays, resilience has come to mean an ability to confront adversity and still find hope and meaning in life."

(Deveson, 2003, p. 6)

Research from the last decade indicates that resilience theory can add to our understanding of how people survive shocking childhood circumstances and continue to develop through their life span (Werner & Smith, 1992; Higgins, 1994; Lifton, 1993; Meirer, 1995). Various factors have been identified as contributing to resilience among those suffering deprivations and hardships, especially as children, but there is general agreement that individuals have the capacity to transform, change, and adapt in unexpected ways to detrimental circumstances. Protective factors (Rak & Patterson, 1966) include personal characteristics, early nurturing, self-concept factors, and supports in the environment. Environmental factors have also been described as an emphasis on collectivity, shared concern, and responsibility for others (Daly, Jannings, Beckett, & Leashore, 1995, quoted in

Shulman, 1999, p. 69). These characteristics were soon identified as existing among the Former British Child Migrant women since childhood

Janoff-Bulman and Timko (1987) suggest that there can also be positive gains from negative experiences earlier in life: "the benefits derived from negative events include a new-found appreciation of life and a recognition of what is really important, as well as a more positive view of one's own possibilities and strengths" (p. 155). Shulman (1999, p. 67) states that "not all children exposed to high degrees of risk and trauma had negative developmental outcomes in their lives," while Louise Bailey writes, "it never ceases to amaze me what people can endure and live through, and it is astounding to see them positively process an event that has changed their lives forever" (Bailey, 1996, p. 23). Werner and Smith (1992) who followed children born into extremely high risk environments found that 50% to 70% grew up to be competent, caring persons.

In the field of aging, Staudinger, Marsiske and Baltes (1993) looked at resilience over the life span and felt that "development throughout life is characterized by joint occurrence of increases (gains), decreases (losses) and maintenance (stability) in adaptive capacity" (p. 542). Resources that can be activated or increased strengthen the positive aspects of the older person's life both internally and externally. Social networks are listed as part of the external positive "reserve capacity" leading to increased resilience throughout the lifespan and Bernard's research (1991) indicated that mentors and teachers could contribute significantly to resilience.

The group of girls who entered Goodwood Orphanage had traveled together for months across the world. Most of them had not known each other when they left England but by Australia they were a surrogate family and continued that way for their years in the institution. They were identified as "different" from the other Australian girls and clung to each other for support, comfort, and connection to the "home" they had lost. Even after leaving the orphanage and starting families of their own they had some knowledge of most of their friends and were available for crisis assistance. The resilience nurtured in each of them was aided by the strong links they made to each others' lives.

An example of this closeness is seen by the fact that there has consistently been a core of five regular members of the group with others coming to various event or meetings. But everyone in the network knows of the activities and many more join in for various events especially those involving public recognition of their experiences. Joys of family reunification are celebrated and tragedies mourned together. In offering services to the core group we are always aware that a broader community is also involved.

THEIR TRAUMA

"The absolute powerlessness and helplessness in trauma cannot be grasped, integrated, or mediated through the human capacity for symbolization."

(LaMothe, 1999, p. 1195)

Greenacre (1952) defined trauma in children as "any condition which seems definitely unfavourable, noxious or drastically injurious to their development" (p. 10) while Herman (1992, p. 96) states that "repeated trauma in adult life erodes the structure of the personality already formed, but repeated trauma in childhood forms and deforms the personality." Although there are many other definitions of trauma (Matsakis 1966; Figley, 1988; Valent, 1998) this one fits well for a group of young children who were uprooted from their homeland and taken with little knowledge of their destination to be placed in an institution, Goodwood Orphanage, that they describe as harsh and uncaring.

They gave numerous examples of their treatment at Goodwood Orphanage, and following are some of the experiences they described. Having been told in England that they were going to be adopted by families in Australia, the children arrived at the orphanage with little preparation for their new lives. As soon as they arrived, their clothes and all personal belongings, including toys, were taken from them. Subsequently, if the children received toys from friends they had made on the boat or families they visited for short periods, these were immediately confiscated.

The children immediately had their hair cut very short, which the older girls found extremely stressful since they had been encouraged by their carers in England to take pride in their hair. These older girls also worked in the laundry for long hours and missed much important time for their education. School for all children was held in the orphanage so that contact with the outside community was limited.

Discipline was very strict with capital punishment freely administered. Harsh physical striking around the face and head was common as was the deprivation of food for misbehaviors. Bed wetters were made to stand with urine stained sheets around their shoulders and a common practice to deter bed wetting was to be hit a child on the buttocks while in bed. The women talked about sometimes waking up to such a thrashing and being afraid to go to sleep in case it happened that night. One of the women told about being stripped naked in front of all the orphanage girls at 14 years of age and hit over her entire body to the extent that she could not sit comfortably for days.

The abuse did not stop at the orphanage because some of the girls were sent at the young ages of 14 or 15 to isolated rural farms where there were few women. Several of these girls were raped or beaten or both. If such acts were reported to the orphanage no action was taken and the girls were left thinking that they were not believed or that what happened was their fault. Those who had not been sent away had to leave the orphanage at 16 and were turned out into the world with no supervision or community support. Over time many appalling and inhuman acts were recalled and attributed to the nuns in charge of the orphanage by the women attending the group meetings at the Loss and Grief Centre. Similar events were reported to the Senate inquiry into the British Child Migrants (Commonwealth of Australia, 2001).

The traumatic experiences the women experienced as children have impacted on all aspects of their subsequent lives and influenced their self confidence, their careers, their educational opportunities, their relationships, their parenting, their expectations in life, and their self concepts. LaMothe (1999) writes about the inability to adequately convey to others the deepest aspect of personal trauma if it is inflicted by another human being, which he believes is essentially different than other kinds of trauma. "The core aspect of the trauma remains non-integrated because the absence of obligation, trust and fidelity in human relations is something that is experienced but cannot be symbolized" (p. 1205). Harvey and Weber add, "we want to emphasize that people can never totally achieve resolution for some major losses" (1998, p. 327).

It was obvious that the women who told narratives of their early experiences were still bearing scars and still feeling strong emotions about what had happened to them and often spoke as if they felt that something irretrievable had been lost. At the same time they exhibited great resilience through their accomplishments such as forming meaningful partnerships, raising children, helping each other, recovering from hospitalization due to emotional illness, seeking counselling, and above all, exerting monumental efforts to locate their families of origin in England. During their work together at the Loss and Grief Centre these two expressions of resilience and trauma were constantly demonstrated.

INITIAL ACTIVITIES: LOSS AND GRIEF AROUND STOLEN IDENTITIES

"There is a growing awareness and theoretical interest in the relationship between bereavement and other kinds of losses, such as dispossession felt by Indigenous people and refugees, or losses associated with adoption."

(Kellehear, 2002 p. 178)

In the process of becoming better acquainted with the group members and gaining trust, gentle activities were constructed that allowed for and encouraged the recognition and naming of the reality of their suffering as children. At the first two meetings a list was constructed of the losses experienced by the women from their forced migration and this list stayed prominently displayed and served as an important reality symbol to what had been lost through the forced migration. Patricia Weenolsen (1988) defines loss as "anything that destroys some aspect, whether macroscopic or microscopic, of life and self" (p. 19) and from her research with women who had encountered intense and varied situations of loss she looks at the layers of loss that follow the initial event or the primary loss. The secondary loss is the immediate effects that follow from the event itself but subsequently holistic, self-conceptual, and metaphorical losses describe how self image, ideas of place in the world, and more abstract meanings are attached to the initial experience (Weenolsen, 1988, p. 55).

Everyone participated in the detailing of their losses and acknowledged the power of the pain around their experiences. The idea of layers of loss seemed helpful in looking deeper into the interpersonal effects of the forced migration. At the end of the first year of the group several women attended the annual Christmas Memorial Service held at the Centre to reflect on and express their deep-seated, longstanding sadness at some past experiences of their lives. The following is the list that was compiled by the group.

LOSSES EXPERIENCED IN THEIR CHILDHOOD

- Abandonment of their birth parents
- Loss of their "home" institution where most reported being treated with respect and care
- Loss of familiar and loved carers
- Loss of foster "aunts" and "uncles" they had in England
- Loss of a carefree attitude and happy activities and innocence
- Loss of community school life they had known in England
- Loss of family in England, parents, siblings, grandparents, extended family

- Loss of possibility for connection to family
- Loss of sense of belonging – being the same as others
- Loss of connection to their childhood experiences
- Being told untruths about their adoption prospects
- Waiting in cages at the docks in England when they were leaving
- Loss of country of birth and recognition as a citizen with rights
- Loss of British culture and British accent
- Loss of trust in adults in their lives
- Loss of personal identity as a child in Britain
- Loss of personal belongings and toys from England
- Loss of dignity

Looking at their experiences through a loss framework was a new perspective to most of the women but it made immediate sense to them. As children there seemed to have been no recognition of the sense of loss or the sadness that was being experienced by these young migrants. They were expected to be grateful for the chance to have a new life in Australia and felt that they had never been allowed to mourn for their lost families, country and birthright. Their grief appeared to have been "disenfranchised" (Doka, 1993), that is, not recognized as legitimate.

> *"There are circumstances in which a person experiences a sense of loss but does not have a socially recognized right, role, or capacity to grieve. In these cases, the grief is disenfranchised. The person suffers a loss but has little or no opportunity to mourn publicly."*

(Doka, 1993, p. 128)

In every interaction and at every meeting of the group the grief of past experiences was acknowledged, and this has remained one of the most important helping responses to the women. As Herman (1992) states, "When the truth is finally recognised, survivors can begin their recovery" (p. 1).

Neimeyer (1998) sees the recovery from grief as the ability to create new meanings after the experience of loss: "meaning reconstruction in response to a loss is the central process in grieving" (p. 338). To a large extent it appeared that such reconstruction had happened through the resilience of the women, their lasting friendships, and their attempts to help each other to survive what had happened to them. But formalizing activities that directly acknowledged the depth of feeling they still carried within, as well as recognizing their courage in the face of such hardship, contributed to creating new meanings in relation to seeing themselves as "victors" over past events.

These early sessions of the group were tentative and involved various members coming and leaving, some home visits, some individual counselling, and some phone conversations, but always a monthly meeting with food and sharing. It was often the case at the meeting that conversation seemed related only to ordinary everyday events that any group of women might discuss. However, never a meeting passed without some recounting of an event or incident from the orphanage, and when that happened each woman joined in with a deeply personal perspective on the subject matter. The depth of the hurt that still remained and that stood along side the resilience was disturbing and at times shocking and indeed it seemed as if LaMothe (1999) was speaking of this group when he said, "Many people who have survived trauma carry a sense of estrangement and burden long after the event" (p. 1203).

SOCIAL JUSTICE THROUGH PUBLIC RECOGNITION

"Letting go of hatred and a desire for revenge does not necessarily open the way for complete forgiveness – not unless there has been a true apology."

(Deveson, 2003, p. 120)

Each month as the group met together they worked on constructing a banner that had been requested by the Migration Museum in Adelaide to be hung in their gallery. As a preparation for this project, a session was held with an artist who asked the women to draw pictures blindfolded and then look at and discuss their drawings. Each person had portrayed a symbol of their traumatic childhood in a most incredible and clearly identifiable manner. The pictures they had drawn were considered very meaningful to the women and most of them saved what they had created. Many of these symbols were incorporated into the banner and the design, selection of materials, drawing of figures and stitching of fabric over many months gave occasion to documenting artistically their past and to expressing their grief collectively.

"A person may write, tell a story, or paint or sculpt their experience of the traumatic event, yet there is something, some black hole that remains outside of symbol and language."

(La Mothe, 1999, p. 1205)

While they were cutting, stitching, or designing, a theme that kept recurring in conversation was the force that the rupture from homeland still had on them even after 50 years. There seemed to be another layer of inner core experiences that remained unidentified or unexpressed, erupting in anger at the church and society for allowing their past to happen at all. The Aboriginal Health Council in South Australia in partnership with the Dulwich Centre has written about the link between social justice and grief (1995, p. 15) stating that "it is much more difficult for people to deal with the effects of grief and loss if the injustices involved are not named." It may be impossible to relinquish grief that has been caused by social injustice until some of that injustice has been addressed and acknowledged. The connection seemed to resonate with the situation of the Former British Child Migrants, and tentatively suggestions were made about moving to activities that brought the past to public attention and acknowledgement.

There was an immediate and enthusiastic response and the oldest member of the group who always felt responsible for the younger girls as children and who now acted as the informal leader and spokesperson of the group took up the reins. Intermingled with conversations about the brutality of the early experiences, plans began for a range of activities aimed at identifying responsibility, gaining public recognition, and seeking apologies.

The State government of South Australia had responded to the publicity about the Former British Child Migrants by placing a plaque in their honor at the South Australian Museum in February of 2001. The dedication was attended by many women who had lived at Goodwood Orphanage and it was an important beginning to public recognition. However, the wording of the statement read at the dedication still left ambiguity about the credibility of the hardships that were endured.

> *"The Government of South Australia wishes to acknowledge that these experiences, though not intended by the schemes, may have occurred and been suffered by the child migrants."*

> (Commonwealth of Australia, 2001, Appendix 7)

The use of the word "may" caused hurt and anger and verified the disenfranchised nature of the grief that had resulted from life in the orphanage. Together the women in the group began a series of activities that sought formal acknowledgement of what had happened to them and formal apologies from the parties concerned. The Australian Commonwealth Senate Community Affairs Reference Committee was conducting interviews with former British Child Migrants as part of their inquiry into what had happened to unaccompanied young children from England. Using support from family and friends several group members came forth to make statements (Commonwealth of Australia, 2001). This was described as stressful and daunting. However, the inquiry also acted as a catalyst to action.

Under the leadership of the woman who acted as the group spokesperson a report was given at each meeting on the month's activities and plans for further actions. Over the next two and a half years these included:

- A series of letters to the Catholic Archbishop explaining the history and asking for a meeting;
- Letters to the Minister for Social Justice asking for an appointment;
- A meeting with a lawyer to discuss legal implications of the most obviously illegal events such as rape;
- Several meetings with the social worker from the British Child Migrant Trust around services available to them;
- A meeting with a representative from the Catholic Church in England who was offering help with finding family members;
- Several meetings with the South Australian Dept of Human services, Adoption and Family Information Service around gaining their assistance for services and a memorial statue;
- Continued work on the banner for the Migration Museum with contribution to this project obtained from the Department of Human Services;
- A meeting with the Minister for Social Justice, which was attended by a large number of women who were articulate in personally expressing their current needs;
- Gaining of funds for continuing education and some housing assistance, resulting from the meeting with the Minister for Social Justice; and
- A project to raise funds for constructing a statue in commemoration of the unaccompanied British Child Migrants. Several meetings were held with the sculptor and a design was selected, of a statue of children standing alone with suitcases. The Australian Federal Government contributed $17,000.00 to this project. Meetings were held with the director of the Migration Museum who applied for and received approval to have the statue placed in the museum garden.

In December of 2001 the Catholic Archbishop agreed to meet the leader of the group with one of the social workers and requests were made for:

- Access to the historical documents and records still held by the church pertaining to the women at the Goodwood Orphanage;
- An apology from the church for the past injustices;
- An acknowledgement of the negative and erroneous portrayal of the British Child Migrants in a book written about the history of the Mercy Sisters in Australia (McLay, 1996); and
- A service of reconciliation.

In addition to this incredible list of activities a wonderful project was conducted in 2003 that was very meaningful to those involved. The life stories of five of the women who were regular group members were compiled with the help of three Master of Social Work students and copies were shared with the group members. Funding was received to put these stories into a more substantial and public book which will be displayed and sold in the Migration Museum. The women expressed the opinion that it was a very significant and validating experience to have their early lives documented and an opportunity to pass on their story to their children and grandchildren. Some family members had not been aware of the past history and were very moved by what they read.

"We share stories to try to understand the lives we have lived, to provide narrative order and coherence to the chaotic disorder and fragmented living that we experience in epiphanies, and to create a life we can live with and a world we can live in."

(Nin, quoted in Ellis, 1998, p. 49)

THE JOURNEY CONTINUES

Travelling as social workers on the road with those who have suffered unjustly and had the courage to survive and construct meaningful lives is a humbling experience. My coworker and myself have contributed our skills and knowledge to their efforts, being careful to respect their pace and direction. Changes have occurred and with each step towards recognition, acknowledgement, and an apology, recovery is strengthened. No one seems to feel that the hurt can be eradicated any more than the innocence of childhood can be reclaimed. But the recovery continues helped by a focus on the loss, grief, and trauma in combination with actions directed at claiming social justice from the society and organizations who so cruelly wounded these women as young children. Our aim always is to build on the resilience that is present in whatever form in each woman and to share our skills and knowledge in this effort, keeping in mind Shulman's comments,

> *"When the social worker represents to the client a professional who believes in the client's capacities for growth, change and adaptation, the social worker becomes one of the sources for resilience in the life of the client."*

(Shulman, 1999, p. 73)

REFERENCES

Aboriginal Health Council of South Australia. (1995). Aboriginal Deaths in Custody: Placing Counselling in a Social Justice Framework. In *Reclaiming Our Stories, Reclaiming Our Lives*. Adelaide: *Dulwich Centre Newsletter*, 1, 2–22.

Bailey, L. (1996). How to Impact Trauma. *Psychotherapy in Australia, 3*(1), 19–23.

Bernard, B. (1991). *Fostering Resiliency In Kids: Protective Factors In The Family, School And Community*. Portland, OR: Northwest Regional Educational Laboratory.

Boss, P. (1999). *Ambiguous Loss: Learning to Live with Unresolved Grief*. Boston: Harvard University Press.

Commonwealth of Australia, (2001). *Lost innocents: Righting the Record*: Report on Child Migration. Canberra, Australian Capital Territory: Senate Community Affairs Reference Committee.

Deveson, A. (2003). *Resilience*. Crows Nest, NSW: Allen and Unwin.

Doka, K. (1993). Disenfranchised Grief: A Mark Of Our Time. In Wandarna Coowar: Hidden Grief, *Proceedings of the Eighth National Conference*. Yappoon, QLD: National Association for Loss and Grief.

Ellis, C. (1998). Exploring Loss Through Autoenthnographic Inquiry: Autoethnographic Stories, Co-Constructed Narratives, And Interactive Interviews. In J. Harvey (Ed.), *Perspectives on Loss* (pp. 49–61). Philadelphia: Brunner/Mazel.

Figley, CR. (1988). *Traumatology and Grieving*. Philadelphia: Brunner/Mazel.

Greenacre, P. (1952). *Trauma, Growth and Personality*. New York: WW Norton.

Harvey, J., and Weber, A. (1998). Why Must There be a Psychology of Loss. In J. Harvey (Ed.), *Perspectives on Loss* (pp. 319–329). Philadelphia: Brunner/Mazel.

Herman, J. (1992). *Trauma and Recovery*. New York: Basic Books.

Higgins, G. (1994). *Resilient Adults: Overcoming a Cruel Past*. San Francisco: Jossey Bass.

Humphries, M. (1994). *Empty Cradles: One Woman's Fight to Uncover Britain's Most Shameful Secrets*. London: Doubleday.

Janoff-Bulman, R., & Timko, C. (1987). Coping with Traumatic Life Events: The Role of Denial in Light of People's Assumptive World. In C. R. Snyder & C. E. Ford (Eds.), *Coping with Negative Life Events* (pp. 135–155). New York: Viking.

Kellehear, A. (2002). Grief and Loss: Past, Present and Future. *Medical Journal of Australia, 177*, 176.

LaMothe, R. (1999). The Absence of Cure. *Journal of Interpersonal Violence, 14*(11), 1193–1210.

Lifton, R. (1994). *The Protein Self: Human Resilience in an Age of Fragmentation.* New York: Basic Books.

Matsakis, A. (1996). *Vietnam Wives: Facing the Challenges of Life with Veterans Suffering Post Traumatic Stress* (2nd ed.). Sydney: The Sidran Press.

McLay, A. (1996). *Women on the Move—Mercy's Triple Spiral.* Adelaide, South Australia: Gillingham Printers.

Mirsky, J. (1991). Language in Migration: Separation Individuation Conflicts in Relation to the Mother Tongue and the new Language. *Psychotherapy, 28*(4), 618.

Neimeyer, R. (1998). Can there be a Psychology of Loss? In J. Harvey (Ed.), *Perspectives on Loss* (pp. 331–341), Philadelphia: Brunner/Mazel.

Rak, C. F, & Patterson, L.E. (1966). Promoting Resilience in at Risk Children. *Journal of Counseling and Development, 74*, 368–373.

Sherington, G., & Jeffery, C. (1998). *Fairbridge: Empire & Child Migration.* Nedlands: University of Western Australia Press.

Shulman, L. (1999). *Skills of Helping Individuals and Groups* (4th ed.). Itasca, IL: F.E. Peacock.

Smith, C., & Carlson, B.E. (1997). Stress, Coping and Resilience in Children and Youth. *Social Service Review*, June, 231–256.

Senate Community Affairs References Committee, (2001) Lost Innocents: Righting the Record. *Report on Child Migration*, Canberra: Senate Printing Unit, Parliament House.

Staudinger, U.M., Marsiske, M., & Baltes, P.B. (1993). Resilience and Levels of Reserve capacity in Later Adulthood: Perspectives from Life-Span Theory. *Development and Psychopathology, 5*(4), 541–566.

Valent, P. (1998). *From Survival to Fulfillment: A Framework for the Life-Trauma Dialectic.* Philadelphia: Brunner/Mazel.

Weenolsen, P. (1988). *Transcendence of Loss Over the Life Span.* New York: Hemisphere.

Werner, E., & Smith, R. (1992). *Overcoming the Odds: High-risk Children from Birth to Adulthood.* New York: Cornell University Press.

Psychiatry, Testimony, and Shoah: Reconstructing the Narratives of the Muted

Baruch Greenwald, MSW
Oshrit Ben-Ari, MSW
Rael D. Strous, MD
Dori Laub, MD

INTRODUCTION

Out of a group of about 5,000 long-term psychiatric patients hospitalized in Israel since 1999, a disproportionate number of about 725 were identified as Holocaust survivors (Bazak Commission, 1999). A review of these cases showed that these patients had not been treated as a unique group, and that their trauma-related illnesses had been neglected in their decades-long treatment. Most of these patients had been diagnosed as having chronic schizophrenia, with no special attention given to the historical circumstances related to their psychiatric symptoms and disabilities. Many of the psychiatrists that treated them insist today that these patients do not respond to traditional treatment such as antipsychotic medication (Cahn, 1995; Riess, 2002). We postulated that many of them could have avoided lengthy if not lifelong psychiatric hospitalization had they been able or had an opportunity in their careers, or by society at large, to more openly share their severe history of persecution. Instead, those gruesome and traumatic experiences remained encapsulated and split off, causing the survivor to lead a double life. These patients may physically inhabit the world as geriatrics, though emotionally they may remain fixed in adolescence. Thus, the aim of this study was to investigate the role of video testimony as a potential useful clinical intervention many years after the acute traumatic event and to analyze the content of the video testimony for clinical material which may be useful in the psychotherapeutic process with the patient.

METHOD

Study Population

The study population consisted of chronic inpatients at two large state referral institutions in Israel. The subjects were drawn from the approximately 100 residents (age range of 59–97 years) housed in the hostel section for Holocaust survivors established in 2000, all of whom have severe, chronic mental illness. For study inclusion, subjects met criteria as victims of Nazi persecution as defined by the Conference on Jewish Claims Against Germany, Inc. (in hiding, ghettos, concentration labor, and death camps etc.), who were at least 3 years old during the time of persecution, and who were willing and capable of telling a story. Survivors were excluded if they exhibited features of major cognitive impairment or severe psychotic disorganization that would preclude video testimony participation. The study was approved by the local Helsinki Committee Ethical Review Committee and the Yale Human Investigation Committee. Subjects and their legal guardians provided signed informed consent once the nature of the study and its potential risks and benefits were fully explained. Consent was also obtained from the subject's designated clinician. In addition to the right to terminate participation at any time during the study, subjects were informed they had the right to prohibit the sharing of video testimony and to withdraw it at any time from the Video Archive or the locked collections for future medical training and research.

Video Testimony

For the purposes of documenting and studying these experiences, 26 patients were recruited and interviewed by mental health professionals. Their testimonies were recorded on videotape. In addition to the video testimony, they also participated in a psychiatric evaluation and psychological testing. By videotaping testimonies of these patients' experiences before, during, and after World War II, we created highly condensed texts that could be interpreted on multiple levels going far beyond the mere narrative content of clinical medical history. We believed that severe psychological trauma could be better addressed through the medium of video testimony. Joint observation, reiteration, and discussion of these testimonies with staff members and the patients, themselves, have proven to be an interesting and important experience. This has been accomplished by means of an individual one by one careful and precise analysis of form and content of the clinical interview.

We have addressed the issue of whether or not massive psychic trauma is related to severe chronic mental illness with a psychotic disability that leads to chronic or multiple psychiatric hospitalizations. For example, patients that had been diagnosed for years as suffering from schizophrenia might have been more correctly diagnosed as having posttraumatic stress disorder (PTSD), which was related to their World War II experiences, and had this been the case, the entire course of treatment might have been altered. Although we know that this diagnostic entity (PTSD) was not in existence as such in the 1950s and 1960s, know-how about PTSD symptoms was already commencing at this time and the diagnostic entity itself has been in the DSM for over 20 years. Likewise, we questioned whether a therapeutic intervention such as a video testimony, which helps build a narrative for the traumatic experience and gives it coherent expression, might help in alleviating the symptoms of the disorder and thus change its course. Whether these changes may be attributed to direct intervention through the patient's testimony or are a result of an indirect intervention through planning treatment, involvement with family members or the survivor community, or the knowledge that the videotaped testimony will be made available to others, is an open question.

During the course of each of the 26 testimony interviews, emphasis was placed on a cooperative reconstruction of a continuous life history containing pre-Holocaust experiences entrapped sometimes in a vague, ambiguous past, a description of the patients' own subjective Holocaust experience, post-World War II experiences until the present, and an attempt to understand what significant role the patients' tragic past plays in their life today. Through this reconstruction, the mourning process is able to take place and hopefully be alleviated. In the years of turmoil and upheaval following World War II, there was often no opportunity to be involved in such a mourning process. The patients were involved in immigrating to a new country (often illegally), fighting for survival, trying to rebuild families, and learning vocations. If one desired to share with others details of their misfortunate past and degrading experiences, neither the layperson nor professional would legitimatize then what we would view today as a therapeutic as well as a humane necessity. Their experiences were too horrendous for members of today's society to absorb. During the testimony interview, steps had to be taken to aid the subjects in restoring that very sense of self that had been dealt such a devastating blow in both the Holocaust and the upheaval thereafter. In the testimony interviews, we attempt to create a narrative that is both detailed and organized, by utilizing cognitive, affective, and sensory elements. The cognitive channel emphasizes a detailed reconstruction of historical facts related to the traumatic events, the affective channel reconstructs feelings then and now, and the sensory channel reconstructs bodily sensations, sights, smells, and sounds. The testimonial experience is a collaborative venture, since the interviewer assumes the position of a companion or compassionate chronicler of a journey into the self and into the past, a journey without any complete pre-existing conscious map of the territory to be uncovered. The document created is intended to be a permanent one for posterity, preserved as a virtual or real record in a safe place. It also serves to affirm facts that the victims either were unable to relate to, or the facts were known but the victims were prevented from telling, or simply did not dare express before the testimonial event.

The video testimony process began with a preliminary impression of the subject's persecution history, gained from either his personal file or a pre-interview, after acquiring permission from the patient and guardian, and responding to any questions and concerns about the subject. A team of two interviewers and a video technician took each testimony. These three individuals were usually outsiders, not previously acquainted with the subjects. Past experience with testimonies have indicated that the victims' pre-existing transference feelings toward people in the interview may impede them in testifying freely and in an unencumbered fashion. The average video session lasted about 60 to 90 minutes. The processed films, which were not edited and contained the contents of the entire sessions, became available to us about six weeks after the initial interviews. After the staff director had viewed the films, individual staff members were invited to sit with the patient and view the testimony together (with the patient's permission). In two cases, the patients objected at first, but agreed later after other patients had finished joint video sessions. The viewing event lasted for one or two sessions, depending on the length of the particular testimony. After the joint viewing, staff members discussed the content with the patient. As a result of these meetings, the staff felt enriched by learning about and vicariously experiencing the patient's life experiences. Consequently, a new and deeper bond was created between the staff and the patients, based on a mutual understanding of the tragic events that played such a major role in the patient's life and pathology. During the joint viewings, we were surprised that a number of the patients could not recognize themselves as the image giving the testimony on the screen. For example, patients said: "Who is that?" or

"How does she know about that? Who told her?" What possible explanations might there be for this phenomenon? Perhaps viewing the images of themselves as encapsulated adolescents conflicted with their present views of themselves and they were unable to understand what had happened to themselves in the intervening years.

Testimonies

While all of the 26 clinical interviews yielded important and fascinating clinical material, the examples of Sarah, David, and Chana (aliases) have been chosen in particular here to illustrate the principal and impact of the testimonial experience. David's silent nature, as well as Sarah's and Chana's general anxiety and fear of leaving the premises of the Holocaust survivor unit could now be viewed in light of severely traumatic events that took place in their early adolescence.

Sarah was born in Greece in 1927, the second of three daughters. A year later, the family was uprooted to Belgium, where her father took a position as Rabbi of a Sephardic community. She had to leave school at the age of 12 and was hidden by others for almost two years in her own home in Nazi-controlled Belgium with her mother and two sisters, who bribed and bartered for survival, only to be eventually turned over to the Nazis by members of the local population and shipped to Auschwitz, where they were separated from their mother, whom they never saw again. The three surviving sisters returned to Belgium after the war, and while attempting to immigrate to Palestine in 1947, they were arrested by the British and held in a camp in Cyprus until they were allowed to immigrate a year later. Arriving in the newborn State of Israel, all three sisters settled on a kibbutz. Sarah describes the death of her older sister from pneumonia, as a result of the severe winter of 1950 (that winter, snow accumulated in most of Israel, the only time in the 20th century). Both of the two remaining sisters married and left the kibbutz for city life. We know of Sarah's subsequent divorce, described by her as a result of her unwillingness to become pregnant and bear children, due to her anxiety. She first began to receive care in a psychiatric outpatient clinic at the age of 34. After her divorce, she lived with her younger sister and her husband and helped care for their three children, until her first hospitalization at age 41 (1968). The reason for her hospitalization was anxiety; the diagnosis was "schizophrenic reaction." Sarah was in and out of several psychiatric hospitals for about three years, after which she was permanently hospitalized. In 1974, at the age of 47, she was sent by the Ministry of Health to a privately run institution. The Ministry opted to close this particular institute toward the end of 1999, after a parliamentary commission investigating the plight of the mentally afflicted Holocaust survivors in Israel found the conditions in this and several other institutions to be appalling (Bazak, 1999). Sarah was then moved to a new Holocaust Survivor Home, not a hospital itself, though located next to the campus of a psychiatric center. The filming of the testimonies took place at the survivor unit. Here are excerpts from Sarah's testimony:

Excerpt 1

Interviewer: Where did they (the Nazis) find you?
Sarah: At home.

I: In your home?

S: Yes, in our home where we hid.

I: Where did you hide in your home?

S: In our own home. They forgot us. They forgot us for two years. Then someone informed them that there were still some Jews in some of the homes. They came to our house, and the first time they let us alone was under the condition that we would never tell anyone they had been there. Two weeks later other Nazis came and took us.

I: Who were the members of your family who hid there?

S: Me, my mother, and my two sisters. I told you, my father had already died of a heart attack. He took all our troubles "to heart" literally. He died on a Friday.

I: Was that after the war began?

S: Yes. You see my father was a Zaddik (righteous man). He got the (heart) attack on Friday (Sabbath eve) and the funeral was on Saturday.

I: Sarah, how were you able to get food while you were hiding in your house?

S: There was a black market. (This) man had a grocery store. It wasn't kosher, but he brought us food we could eat, good stuff. We paid him a lot of money. Thank God my mother had two heavy gold bracelets. She sold them for a lot of money. We were lucky, we bought eggs, yellow cheese, white cheese, jam, and white bread.

I: You paid him and he brought it to your home?

S: Yes, he brought (food) every night.

I: He wasn't a Jew?

S: Of course not, he was a Christian. He brought us food and got paid well for his services. He did it for the money. We were lucky. We had money because my mother sold her jewelry.

I: Where was your hiding place? What did it look like?

S: It was our own home. They forgot us. So we lived.

I: You mean they forgot you because there had already been searches and most of the Jews had been deported?

S: Yes, of course. They forgot us!

I: How was it that they forgot you, wasn't your home near (the other Jewish homes)?

S: No! They had a list of homes, our home was not on the list. They forgot us! That was our luck. If not, we would have been taken with all the others.

I: How did you live your lives in hiding for those two years? What was it like together? How was life during the day, during the night?

S: We lived in constant fear.

I: You were always scared?

S: Yes, we were always scared that they would come and take us. In the end, they were informed and they really did come and get us.

I: Did you ever leave the house (during the two years)?

S: No, never. Can you imagine it? For two years we never left the house. There was always fear that at any second they would come and take us. (sighs) I've been through so much in my life. I was also (imprisoned) in Cyprus.

Excerpt 2

I: How did they find you at home?

S: They were informed. Some children told them in Flemish "There are still some Jews in that house." Can you imagine how we felt? They betrayed us. But still, the first time they came to our house they let us stay, on the condition that we would never tell anyone we had been there. Some of the Belgians were good.

I: Those who came, were they Nazis or Belgians?

S: One was a Nazi, one was a Belgian policeman.

I: Those who came and took you in the end, were they Nazis or Belgians?

S: Nazis, of course.

I: What did they look like?

S: Like Nazis, *Oy Veh* (oh my goodness!). They looked like demons!

I: Were they in uniform?

S: Yes, with swastikas. I saw the same ones at Auschwitz. They came with dogs.

I: Where did they take you?

S: They took us to a police station near Antwerp. There we joined the other groups who were transported to Auschwitz.

I: In trucks?

S: First we were in a jail. Before the trip to Auschwitz. (when they came to our house) they took my mother and sister first. We remained in the house. They told us they would return soon to take us. I asked them if they would let us have coffee. They said, "Coffee will be waiting for you downstairs." I believed them. "Coffee" was the trip to Auschwitz.

I: The Nazi said. "Coffee will be waiting for you." This is important. They cheated you.

S: Yes, and now I will be getting reprimands from Germany. My sister already received them.

I: A truck was there for you downstairs?

S: Yes, they took us (to the station). There we were put on a train. They took us all, standing, in a cattle car. Three days. Three nights. Poor mother. Can you imagine? It was an open cattle car. Three days and three nights till we arrived (at Auschwitz). There they separated us from Mother. We never saw her again.

Many of the staff had not been aware of Sarah's hiding during the war, and even those of us who knew her history were not always aware of the intensity of her experiences during the entire war and thereafter. All we know about Sarah's psychiatric history supports a consistent picture of anxiety related to traumatic experience. Psychiatric testing before her testimony indicated PTSD symptoms. Sarah rarely ventured outside the premises of the Home, and on rare occasions when the staff had succeeded in convincing her to participate in outings, she was tense all the time, even screaming, for example, when the bus hit a bump, or if there were sudden noises. The night staff reported that Sarah still has nightmares about her experiences at Auschwitz. On the premises of the Home, Sarah is an active participant in all activities; she has a tendency to criticize staff members who may not meet all her immediate requests and has developed a dependent, sometimes symbiotic relationship with her roommate. The roommate, a younger woman who was a small child at the end of the Holocaust, grew up as an orphan, and some of her current psychotic content is the delusion that Sarah is really her mother. However, Sarah is not delusional or psychotic today. We think that her 1968 diagnosis of having a "schizophrenic reaction" is dubious and wonder how her life might have changed had she been given more appropriate treatment in the community, with behavioral therapy for anxiety, instead of being hospitalized all her life.

David, born in Czechoslovakia in 1934, was the younger of two siblings. We know that David began elementary school around 1940, already a time of turmoil. It was reported that he was an excellent pupil, very pedantic in his studies. The "normal" life of the family was soon interrupted by the war and the Holocaust, since they were able to survive only by hiding in bunkers for four, perhaps five years. Four years after the war (1949), the family immigrated to Israel, where David completed his high-school matriculation as well as army duty. In the army he had disciplinary problems and was discharged before serving his full term of duty. His first psychiatric hospitalization was in 1957, two years after his discharge from the army. His complaints then included anxiety and somatic symptoms. Like Sarah, he was hospitalized "on and off" in government-run hospitals for several years until he was permanently hospitalized in 1965 at the age of 31 in the same privately run institution that was closed in 1999, when David also moved to the new Holocaust Survivor's Home.

David was a very quiet man who never said more than two or three words. All that we knew about him was from his file or his elderly aunt. At first he refused to participate in the interview. However, soon after he suddenly said: "Okay, let's do it!" He said little and most of the interview consisted of the interviewer speaking, to which he agreed or disagreed. David had no real memories of those years spent in the bunkers, only of asking his mother: "Why are we here?" He can't remember what she answered. When asked whether he felt terror all the time, his answer was, "Probably." His facial and body expressions did speak of terror and sadness, yet he refused to acknowledge that he felt something. David was one of the only patients in the survivor's unit almost constantly silent but prone to violent outbursts if and when he felt his private space had been violated. This silent nature, which perhaps characterizes as many as 20% of the hospitalized psychiatric survivors, has its own uniqueness. These patients seem to walk around, intently observe, smoke, and then unexpectedly walk away. Some seem to be in a conflict or in a struggle when trying to pronounce a word. Even in interviews with many of the survivors that did talk, many deny memories of the Holocaust or simply use code words like "It was awful, you know" or "What is there to talk about?" David also viewed his testimony video together with staff members but had no verbal reactions to the film. Apparently, David had been suffering, and he died unexpectedly four months after his testimony, of massive, undiagnosed lung cancer.

Chana's videotaped testimony was shown at the Fourth International Conference on Social work in Health and Mental Health in Quebec in May, 2004. Chana had agreed to our showing of her film to an overseas audience, yet we have abided by her request not to show it to her son. Interestingly, a day after giving her permission, she appeared in the director's office urgently requesting that a copy of the film remain in Israel should her son wish to view it in the future. We calmed her, explaining that we have two copies of the film, one intended for the researchers and a second one, her copy, which has also remained in our hands at her request. Usually the second copy is given to a guardian or family member after permission from the patient.

Chana was born in a village in eastern Romania in 1927, the youngest child in a family of five siblings. Shortly after the war began, the family was forcibly uprooted and moved to the primarily Jewish town of Yasi. Chana remained in Yasi after the war, wed, bore a child, and divorced, all before immigrating to Israel in 1948. In Israel she lived with her sister and son, wed again, and divorced again after a second son. She was already showing signs of so-called mental illness, and did not raise her second son, with whom she has been separated ever since. From information we have in her file, self-neglect and behavior described as unusual or bizarre preceded psychiatric hospitalizations. Diagnosed as having paranoid schizophrenia, she was in and out of hospitals until the Health Ministry authorized her permanent hospitalization in the same previously mentioned privately run institution in 1980. She also moved to the Holocaust Survivor's Home when the private institution was closed.

Excerpt 1

    Interviewer: Can you remember the massacre of Jews that took place in Yasi?

       Chana: It was. It was. My father buried maybe a thousand victims. He dug a huge pit.

   I: Your father?

   C: (My) father. Dug a huge pit and dropped the bodies. They were naked. They came from the Death Train. Daddy had to take the corpses. I think, I remember I helped him; we put them on a wagon. We carried them to the pit.

   I: In Yasi 30,000 Jews were killed at the beginning (of the war).

C: It was. I forgot how you call it. A massacre.

I: A massacre of the Jews. A huge pogrom. And they called your father to come and help bury (the dead).

C: Yes.

I: They took children (to help bury)?

C: Yes, they took. The Germans came and forced us. They said, "*schneller! schneller!*" (Faster, faster).

I: Can you remember how the Germans looked?

C: I remember how they looked.

I: How did they look?

C: They had green forest uniforms.

I: As a child . . .

C: 12 years old

I: Yes, 12 years old, you yourself already had to bury corpses. How did that affect you?

C: It instilled in me fear. A deep fear. A fear of death. (sighs)

Excerpt 2

C: Suddenly there was an alarm. Airplanes came to bomb us. We did not know whether or not to run to the bunker. I stayed in the house. They all ran to the bunker. We had an old grandmother, mother's mother. My sister took her. I stayed alone in the house. Then the bombing began. I did not know whether or not I should run to the bunker. I was afraid if I stayed in the house it would collapse on me. I did not know what to do. Then I decided to run to the bunker. Shrapnel fell near my leg. I did not know whether to continue running or stay where I was in the middle of the street.

I: So you ran to the bunker?

C: Yes, I ran to the bunker. I did not know what to do, to run or stay where I was. Afterwards a bomb fell (directly) on the second bunker next to us. Everyone was buried; we dug ourselves out with our hands.

I: Everyone was buried?

C: Yes.

I: You were in the bunker when this happened?

C: Yes, I was there.

I: During the bombing?

C: We all sought refuge.

I: The bunker collapsed, but you all got out.

C: (agrees)

Excerpt 3

  C: (sighs) It's hard to remember all of this.

  I: It's hard to remember. Do these pictures come back even when you don't want (to think about it)?

  C: I have dreams about it. But then I realize that, thank God, we are here now, free. It's a great miracle. But they shouldn't throw us out of here as well. I think about it. Maybe they will close down this place and throw us out, who knows where! (pause, then looking straight at the interviewer) Will they close this place?

  I: No, never.

After viewing Chana's testimony in its entirety, the staff members can now more easily recognize the connection between Chana's traumatic childhood, her suspicious behavior, lack of trust, self-neglect, and inability to make independent decisions or even be critical. However, this does not seem to be due to a lack of affect as a negative symptom of schizophrenia. She currently has no delusional behavior. Her psychiatric testing before the testimony indicates both PTSD and some symptoms of psychosis, with a slight decrease in the post-test. What we observe on a daily basis is a sad, older lady, who in the course of her lifetime has experienced uprooting from place to place, mostly unwilling, village to village, country to country, until she reached the Survivor Home. Even at the Survivor Home, she tends to define for herself what she considers as a "safe" territory, often standing at the entrance to her room and leaving only to go to the dining room at meal times or when a staff member calls her for a specific activity. Before the taping of the testimonies, it was known that Chana never attended outings organized by the staff, including concerts, movies, or one-day trips. During 2004, a student, under our close supervision, worked intensely with Chana, making every effort to gain her trust and to get her to join her in attending both inside and outside activities, with only partial success. Unfortunately, the tense security and terror situation in Israel has added to Chana's insecurity. The staff members found her last remarks in the testimony both genuine and sad: "Will they throw us out of here and throw us who knows where?"

CONCLUSIONS

Since we are dealing with patients that have been institutionalized for 20 to 30 years and more, we need to properly characterize them today not only as Holocaust survivors, but also as survivors of psychiatric hospital-ization. As a result, many of these patients have undergone a process of institutionalization and have lost interest in life outside the hospital surroundings. Impressions that we have collected, from both those patients videotaped and those not, support changing the sole diagnosis of schizophrenia, which was assigned for years to many of the mentally afflicted survivors. We may be dealing with a long-term PTSD with psychotic features, in some cases. We are well aware of the fact that survivors previously unable to discuss their traumatic past are now form-ing new bonds with staff members, who, as a result of the survivors' testi-monies, are much more aware of the patients' history. A therapeutic group, using both the contents of the testimonies and other reminiscing techniques, has provided new venues for self-expression, and even the social outings of the patients have now taken on a new significance, since staff members have been able to convince some of the previously immo-bile residents to participate. Knowing and understanding their past has made its impact. Realizing that as a result of the Holocaust trauma, the individual's very sense of self was very often erased, we are attempting to take steps to restore that self, by enabling more self-expression and encouraging empowerment.

REFERENCES

Bazak, Y. (1999), The Findings of the Public Committee of Inquiry into the Situation of the Psychiatrically Ill Patients Hospitalized in Israeli Psychiatric Facilities (Hebrew, available from the Israeli Ministry of Health). The committee was composed of parlia-mentary members, government ministers, and experts in the field.

Cahn, D. (1995), Holocaust Survivors Mistreated, Associated Press release, November 26, 1995.

Rees, M. (2002), Surviving the Past, Time Magazine, January 14, 2002.

Evidence-Based Policy and Social Work in Health and Mental Health

Edward J. Mullen

Harnessing the power of research to achieve treatment targets and to build health systems that respond to the broad array of complex health issues requires an innovative approach to gathering and sharing information. Existing, classic methods of research and dissemination of new knowledge, while still necessary, will not be sufficient to achieve these goals. In the short term, new methods of assessing the performance of treatment programmes are essential. So, too, is the rapid sharing of information in order for countries to benefit from the most recent and most relevant experience elsewhere and adapt it to local circumstances. (World Health Organization, 2004, p. 73)

This article describes how social work can contribute to building a more compassionate and just world with effective and equitable policy, program, and service outcomes in health and mental health, through the use of knowledge, including knowledge derived from experience and research. It proposes that the current emphasis on evidence-based health-care can contribute to the achievement of outcomes that matter to those seeking to build a better world.

CHALLENGES IN THE USE OF KNOWLEDGE FOR HEALTH POLICY

Knowledge is the most valuable resource available to policy makers to achieve improved health and well-being around the world, a fact highlighted in the World Bank's 1999 World Development Report, *Knowledge for Development* (World Bank, 1999). In selecting knowledge as the central policy focus at the turn of the millennium, the World Bank sent an important signal:

> KNOWLEDGE IS LIKE LIGHT. Weightless and intangible, it can eas-ily travel the world, enlightening the lives of people everywhere. Yet billions of people still live in the darkness of poverty - unnecessarily. Knowledge about how to treat such a simple ailment as diarrhea has existed for centuries - but millions of children continue to die from it because their parents do not know how to save them. . . . Better knowl-edge about nutrition can mean better health, even for those with little to spend on food. Knowledge about how to prevent the transmission of AIDS can save millions from debilitationg illness and premature death. Public disclosure of information about industrial pollution can lead to a cleaner and more healthful environment. . . . Knowledge gives people greater control over their destinies. (World Bank, 1999, p. 2)

Knowledge can have dramatic impacts on health. An illustration of the impact of knowledge on health is the case of infant mortality. Infant mor-tality, a key indicator of health worldwide, fell markedly during the last century for all income groups. There remain marked differences based on country per capita income, but much of the reduction in infant mortality cannot be explained by income alone. Increased knowledge accounts for much of the outcome through such efforts as the control of communicable diseases with new drugs, vaccines, and epidemiological knowledge; increased education contributing to adoption and use of health knowledge; and the increased use of information technology to spread medical knowl-edge and sanitary information faster (World Bank, 1999, pp. 17–18).

While the example of infant mortality shows how increased knowledge can have a dramatic impact, the converse is also true. The absence of knowledge can undercut human development and cripple the formulation of intelligent social policies. Nowhere is this more evident than in mental health policy. The World Health Organization's (WHO) *World Health Report 2001* points out that:

> Both the formulation and evaluation of policy require the existence of a well-functioning and coordinated information system for mea-suring a minimum number of mental health indicators. Currently around a third of countries have no system for the annual reporting of mental health data. Those which have such a system often lack sufficiently detailed information to allow for the evaluation of

policy, services and treatment effectiveness. About half the countries have no facilities for the collection of epidemiological or service data at the national level. (pp. 81–82)

The WHO report underscores the crippling effect on social policies and programs when knowledge is absent. While health research has generated a great deal of knowledge and technology, the report notes that "there still remain many unknown variables which contribute to the development of mental disorders, their course and their effective treatment" (World Health Organization, 2001, p. 104). The report calls for more research "to help better understand the epidemiology of mental disorders, and the efficacy, effectiveness and cost-effectiveness of treatments, services and policies" (p. 104).

Perhaps the greatest current knowledge gap in health and mental health is the absence of culturally informed research. Much of the knowledge that has been developed in health and mental health has come from the developed countries. Yet, this knowledge as well as the methods and tools used to develop it cannot be assumed to fit the culture and circumstances of other countries, especially the developing countries that are the poorest. As the WHO report notes: "In many developing countries there is a notable lack of scientific research on mental health epidemiology, services, treatment, prevention and promotion, and policy" (World Health Organization, 2001, p. 106). Knowledge, when it is available and effectively disseminated and absorbed, can have dramatic effects on the improvement of population health. Conversely, when this is not the case, crippling effects can result, since without information, reasonable decision making is undercut. And, even when knowledge is available, if it is not culturally relevant its utility is lessened and, indeed, harm can result. In the absence of culturally relevant knowledge there is "no rational basis to guide advocacy, planning and intervention" (World Health Organization, 2001, p. 106). The problem is that there are major inequities in the distribution of knowledge. The challenge is not only to foster the continued development of knowledge but also to find better ways of getting available knowledge to populations in need—such as through better use of information and communication technology—and helping populations develop a capacity for proper use of such knowledge, such as, for example, by providing primary education. Large segments of the world, especially the poorest of the developing countries, simply lack access to or the capacity to use the knowledge that is already available. As the World Bank report notes: "Poor countries—and poor people—differ from rich ones not only because they have less capital but because they have less knowledge" (World Bank, 1999, p. 1).

Health policies are based on many factors in addition to knowledge, including politics, resources, self-interests, values, and ideologies. Knowledge use for population health and mental health betterment, even when it exists in usable form, can be undercut by politics. As the WHO report notes:

> One lesson of the past 50 years is that tackling mental disorders involves not only public health but also science and politics. What can be achieved by good public health policy and science can be destroyed by politics. If the political environment is supportive of mental health, science is still needed to advance understanding of the complex causes of mental disorders, and to improve their treatment. (World Health Organization, 2001, p. 106)

POLICY MAKER'S USE OF KNOWLEDGE IN DECISION MAKING

Recent accounts of how knowledge derived from research has been used to formulate policies identify promising strategies as well as significant obstacles (Davies, 2004; Walker, 2001).

Obstacles to the Use of Knowledge for Policy

Obstacles or impediments to the greater use of research are well-known and include the following.

- Policy makers typically work in pressurized environments, needing to deal with immediate issues of the day. There may be little time to search for and to use research systematically when decisions need to be made immediately.
- Often policy decisions are driven primarily by political or organisational self-interest rather than data. The force of values, ideologies and limited resources often overwhelm whatever influence research findings might possibly have.
- Policy makers are often skeptical about the validity of much research because:
    - It is frequently conducted by advocates or contractors who are not independent of funding sources.
    - Research findings are often reported without inclusion of cost analyses which need to be included in policy decisions.

- The research may be of questionable validity pertaining to policy decisions that need to be made. For example, research findings may be based on random controlled trials conducted in highly artificial environments, and therefore, application to specific real-world contexts may be questionable.
- When research is used by policy makers it is often misused to advocate or justify a preferred position.
- Research findings are often used in an ad hoc and post hoc fashion rather than as part of a strategic process. For example, when confronted with a policy issue the policy makers or their staffs may look for studies or reviews that can be plugged into the policy issue at hand. This is very different from systematically using research in the context of a strategic process and in a climate wherein information and knowledge is valued and a part of the decision making culture.
- Busy policy makers don't have the time or, often, the expertise to read lengthy, technical research reports. Researchers have typically not communicated their work in easily-understood brief communications designed for the policy arena.
- Policy making is a process, rather than a discrete point-in-time event. When it comes to national or regional policy decisions many decision makers and interest groups are involved and many people need to be influenced by the research if it is to be used effectively. It is not a matter of using research to influence one person only. Accordingly, if research is to be used, it needs to systematically infuse the process from early on and not be presented solely at the time of the final vote or appropriation.

If research is to be used effectively for policy, these obstacles need to be addressed and significant cultural changes will be required in terms of how the research community conducts and communicates research findings and in terms of how policy groups and organizations manage the knowledge needed to make wise policy decisions.

Using Evidence to Challenge the Cursory Use of Research in Policy

The following episode, recorded in the U.S. *Congressional Record* in 1995, presents a vivid, first-hand account of how social research has been misused in the social policy process, as well as how an astute policy maker, Senator Daniel Patrick Moynihan, can draw upon evidence to correct the situation. The late U.S. Senator and former Harvard University professor, Daniel Patrick Moynihan was a policy maker who was also an astute and well-informed social scientist. J. A. Muir Gray (2001, p. 27) cites Senator Moynihan's congressional testimony as an example of how evidence can be used to alter policy, but the testimony shows much more. It presents a vivid picture of how social science in the best of cases has been used by the likes of Senator Moynihan. Senator Moynihan's testimony was presented in the context of the U.S. congressional debate of 1995 regarding welfare reform. Moynihan is presenting an argument against funding a new program called Family Preservation which was to provide intensive social services to families at risk of having a child placed out of the home. As part of his testimony he placed into the U.S. *Congressional Record* a letter he had written to Dr. Laura D'Andrea Tyson, then the Chairman of the Council of Economic Advisors (July 28, 1993). The excerpt from Moynihan's letter to Tyson shows how evaluation research findings were used in this congressional funding debate.

> Dear Dr. Tyson: You will recall that last Thursday when you so kindly joined us . . . you and I discussed the President's family preservation proposal. You indicated how much he supports the measure. I assured you I, too, support it, but went on to ask what evidence was there that it would have any effect. You assured me there was such data. . . . I asked for two citations. The next day we received a fax from . . . your staff with a number of citations and a paper. . . . The paper is quite direct: "solid proof that family preservation services can effect a state's overall placement rates is still lacking. . . . Overall, the Family First placement prevention program results in a slight increase in placement rates. . . ." In other words, there are either negative effects or no effects . . . there is nothing the least surprising in either of these findings[.] From the mid-'60s on this has been the repeated, I almost want to say consistent pattern of evaluation studies. Either few effects or negative effects. . . . In the last six months, I have been repeatedly impressed by the number of members of the [President's] Administration who have assured me with great vigor that something or other is known in an area of social policy which, to the best of my understanding, is not known at all. (Congressional Record, pp. S18434–S18435)

Senator Moynihan's letter illustrates a number of important points about how social research has often been used in policy debates. First, research can be used to justify or to discredit a previously held position. Second, studies can be cited but the evidence may not be examined closely, or at all, until there is a challenge. Third, findings may be used and cited in an ad hoc fashion or out of context.

Misuse of Evidence by Failing to Consider Unintended Negative Social Consequences

There are many examples of how advances in knowledge and technology are used by policy makers but without consideration being given to possible negative effects. This type of usage can be considered misuse, jumping to conclusions without careful consideration of consequences. A further story narrated by Senator Moynihan and recorded in the U.S. *Congressional Record* illustrates this misuse. It is well known that remarkable advances in psychopharmacology research beginning in the 1950s made it possible to control psychotic symptoms and behaviors sufficiently to consider community care, rather than custodial institutional care, for the severely mentally ill. Accordingly, in the United States, there was a mass closing of mental hospitals beginning in the 1950s in large part made possible by these advances in psychopharmacological research. However, inadequate attention and resources were put into the necessary community supports required. This is an example of how medical research findings and technological developments can be misused when social policies are not developed sufficiently to accommodate the social consequences of such technological advances. Moynihan gives a pointed account of how this happened in New York State.

> I have frequently referred to the Federal legislation that commenced the deinstitutionalization of mental patients. . . . Early in 1955 . . . Jonathan B. Bingham, at that time secretary to Governor Averell Harriman of New York brought Dr. Paul Hoch, the new commissioner of mental health, in to meet the Governor. I was present, along with Paul H. Appleby, the new budget director. Dr. Hoch, a wonderful, humane man of science, told of a new chemical treatment for mental illness which had been developed by Dr. Nathan Kline at Rockland State Hospital in the lower Hudson Valley. It had been tested clinically. Hoch proposed that it be given to all patients, throughout the New York mental hospital system, which then held some 94,000 patients. Today [in 1995] there are 8,000. Harriman asked what the program would cost. Hoch mentioned a sum in the

neighborhood, as I recall, of $4 million. Harriman asked Appleby if he could find the money. Appleby . . . replied that he could find it. Done. said Harriman, I am an investment banker and believe in investment. And so reserpine medication commenced. Eight years later, on October 22, 1963 . . . President John F. Kennedy signed the Community Health Center Construction Act of 1963. . . . We were going to empty out our great mental hospitals and treat patients in local community centers. We would build 2,000 by the year 1980, and thereafter one for each additional 100,000 persons in the population. Alas, we built some 400 centers, and then just forgot about our earlier plans. But we emptied out the hospitals. A decade or so later, the problem of the homeless appeared, to our general bafflement. (U.S. Congressional Record, p. S18436–S18437)

This account from Senator Moynihan illustrates vividly how advances in knowledge and technology can result in dire social consequences if not carefully thought through and especially if social policies are not carefully considered, in this case how to create a sustainable, compassionate and just community environment for the seriously mentally ill once the institutions were closed.

As these examples show there are many challenges and barriers in the policy process to the proper and constructive use of knowledge especially that based on scientific research. Nevertheless, research has and no doubt will continue to influence policy in significant ways. The challenge is to find better ways to bring knowledge, including that derived from scientific research, into the policy process.

KNOWLEDGE USE FOR POLICY AS A 21ST CENTURY CHALLENGE

Knowledge creation, diffusion, and utilization as an area of study and application was extensively developed in the last half of the 20th century (Rich, 1978). However, because of recent developments, this topic has been transformed because of the rapid expansion of knowledge and information technology as well as the globalization of knowledge and information. In addition, there has been a massive and rapid development of informed citizens in many of the world's countries, such that more and more citizens are coming to health services better informed and expecting state of the art health care. Accordingly, in response to these developments new approaches to information and knowledge management are developing which are transforming how policies, programs and services in health and mental health are formulated, implemented and evaluated. These new approaches seek to harness knowledge and information technology and place them in the context of values, resources, citizen preferences, and politics.

Evidence-Based Policy: A Response to 21st Century World Problems and Contexts

In health and mental health the most visible and vigorous of these new approaches is evidence-based healthcare or more broadly evidence-based policy and practice. Because of the many factors that influence the policy and practice process in addition to evidence, and because evidence can play a strong or weak role, some refer to this new approach as evidence-informed practice, or evidence for practice and policy (Grayson & Gomersall, 2003; Nutley, 2003). Sandra Nutley, Isabel Walter and Huw Davies (2002) describe evidence in the context of evidence-based policy as the results of "systematic investigation towards increasing the sum of knowledge" (p. 2). There are differing points of view about what qualifies as systematic investigation (see for example Davies, et al., 2000, chapter 1). Most would agree that the results of controlled experimental research studies would qualify, but there is much debate about how many of the alternative approaches to research should be included as sources of evidence. It is common practice in the evidence-based approaches to include evidence from sources other than controlled research. Reflecting the working definition of evidence used by the U.K. Cabinet Office, Philip Davies (2004, p. 15) cites as sources of evidence: impact evidence; implementation evidence; descriptive analytic evidence; attitudinal evidence; statistical modeling; economic/econometric evidence; and ethical evidence. Accordingly, in the context of evidence-based policy and practice, *evidence* is a type of knowledge that is derived from systematic, empirical analysis of quantitative or qualitative data so as to inform policy or practice decisions.

EVIDENCE-BASED POLICY AND PRACTICE

J. A. Muir Gray (2001), Director of the Institute of Health Sciences at the University of Oxford and among the leading contributors to evidence-based healthcare, has identified problems and pressures on healthcare systems around the world that evidence-based healthcare is responsive to, and can help address. Regarding problems Gray (2001, p. 1) notes that despite the differences in the ways in which health services around the world are funded and organized, many of the major problems in the delivery of healthcare are similar. They include:

- Increasing costs of healthcare, especially due to inflation and ineffi-ciencies.
- Lack of capacity in any country to pay for the totality of health ser-vices demanded by healthcare professionals and the general public.
- Marked variation in the rates of delivery of health services within a country and among countries.
- Delayed implementation of research findings into practice.

Gray (2001, p. 2) places these problems in the context of a worldwide aging of the population, rising citizen expectations, and the growth of new health technology and knowledge. He sees a number of responses to these problems and contexts that are occurring worldwide, including a focus on cost control, efforts to prevent costs from falling on individuals, the growth in importance of the purchasing function focusing on value for money, greater involvement of purchasers in management of practice, and "increasing public and political interest in the evidence on which deci-sions about the effectiveness and safety of healthcare are based" (p. 3). He argues that "In order to meet these powerful challenges, the principles of evidence-based healthcare can be applied to great effect" (p. 3). Drawing on recent experience, Gray notes that pre-conditions must be met for evi-dence-based healthcare including a commitment to cover whole popula-tions and a fixed budget. Under these conditions there is a growing appreciation of the need for evidence-based decision-making.

Doing more good than harm at a reasonable cost is one of the slogans of the evidence-based approach. In the absence of evidence that this is the case, questions can be raised about the wisdom of policies, programs or treatments when resources are scarce. Gray (2001) characterizes evidence-based healthcare as a discipline centered "upon evidence-based decision-making about groups of patients, or populations, which may be manifest as evidence-based policy-making, purchasing or management" (p. 9). He notes that this approach draws evidence from a wide range of disciplines engaged in scientific research, and emphasizes the use of scientific research findings and logic for the analysis of healthcare problems; the identification and appraisal of options for health improvement; and decision-making about the delivery of healthcare for groups of patients or populations (p. vii). This approach to healthcare evolved from work at McMaster University and what is now the Institute of Health Sciences at Oxford University. It was inspired by the earlier work of the McMaster group which resulted in an approach to the treatment of individual patients called evidence-based medicine, defined as the "conscientious, explicit and judicious use of current best evidence in making decisions about the care of individual patients" (Sackett, et al., 1996, p. 71); and the "integration of best research evidence with clinical expertise and patient values" (Sackett, Straus, Richardson, Rosenberg, & Haynes, 2000, p. 1).

The evidence-based medicine approach has rapidly moved into other healthcare professions including social work (Gibbs, 2003; Mullen, 2004a and b; Mullen, Shlonsky, Bledsoe, and Bellamy, 2005; Roberts and Yeager, 2004). The generic form can be referred to as evidence-based clinical practice or simply evidence-based practice. Philip Davies (2004) has described evidence-based policy as an approach that: "helps people make well informed decisions about policies, programmes and projects by putting the best available evidence from research at the heart of policy development and implementation" (p. 3). According to Davies this approach stands in contrast to *opinion*-based policy, which relies heavily on either the selective use of evidence (e.g. on single studies irrespective of quality) or on the untested views of individuals or groups, often inspired by ideological standpoints, prejudices, or speculative conjecture (Davies, 2004, p. 3).

While evidence-based healthcare and evidence-based practice share a common set of assumptions and processes, they target different levels of decision making. Evidence-based practice is focused on individual patients or clients, whereas evidence-based healthcare focuses on groups and populations. The common processes serve to bring about decision making that is based on the best available evidence, sound logic, and involvement of key stakeholders.

EVIDENCE-BASED POLICY STEPS

There are three key steps typically described in an evidence-based approach which I adapt from Gray (2001, pp.xxi-xxiii): (1) finding and appraising the evidence; (2) developing the capacity of individuals and organizations to use the evidence wisely; and, (3) getting the evidence into practice.

Finding and appraising evidence pertaining to the decision at hand includes identification of healthcare options; specifying outcomes of interest such as effectiveness, safety, quality, efficiency, equity; and determining the type of research method to rely on, such as systematic reviews, primary studies, and so forth.

Developing the capacity of organizations and individuals to use evidence involves ensuring that the individual decision makers are capable of practicing evidence-based decision making and seeing to it that organizational structures, cultures, and systems support evidence-based processes.

Getting the evidence into practice involves policy preparation; making cultural changes; and, designing systems for implementation, monitoring, and audit.

In all of these descriptions the evidence-based approach is seen as a decision-making process in which policy-makers, purchasers, managers, or practitioners together with key stakeholders make decisions about problem or need assessment, goals and objectives, interventions and outcomes.

CONCLUDING OBSERVATIONS: GREAT PROMISE BUT A NEED FOR CAUTION

The evidence-based approach has generated much debate (Mullen and Streiner, 2004). Some have seen it as a major new approach applicable to a wide range of disciplines and professions (for example, Marshall, 1995; Sackett, et al., 1997; Gambrill, 1999; Macdonald, 1999; Gibbs & Gambrill, 2002; Gray, 2001). Because of its promise many evidence-based centers have been established around the world and journals and texts are now readily available. Others have criticized evidence-based approaches as threatening professional autonomy and expertise as well as for a variety of other reasons (see for example, Grahame-Smith, 1995; Morgan, 1995; Britton, Evans, & Potter, 1998; Clinicians for the Restoration of Autonomous Practice Writing Group, 2002; Webb, 2001).

The task ahead is to keep clearly in mind the character of the new age, an age where in knowledge and information are powerful resources that can be used to improve global health and mental health. Evidence-based approaches hold great promise for helping to manage this resource effectively. There is no doubt that in the coming decades there well be an increased reliance on knowledge in healthcare including healthcare policy making, purchasing, and management. What forms these new approaches to harnessing the promise of new knowledge and technology will take is unpredictable. Nevertheless, many of the qualities now found in the evidence-based approach will be found to be valuable and deserving of further refinement.

While on first appearance the evidence-based approach seems reasonable, a critical assessment needs to be made as it is rolled out into healthcare. While the approach would seem to have incorporated much of what has been learned over the past half-century about research use for policy and practice, it is new and largely untested. We have seen many promising and innovative strategies for the use of research to improve policy and practice in the past, only to find that there were serious flaws. It is important to be mindful that while we live in an age in which knowledge and information has exploded, the task of using this most valuable resource for the betterment of social policies has not yet been realized. So, we need to be critical about how this innovation will be used and what its outcomes for human development will be in the long run.

While I am confident that the evidence-based policy and practice initiative has much to offer, I am even more convinced that the fundamental challenge is to rethink how best to facilitate the rapid generation, sharing, and application of knowledge in a manner that closes the policy and practice gap. Knowledge needs to be managed much more effectively than it has been in the past. Nowhere is this more apparent than in the current HIV/AIDS pandemic. I conclude as I began with a quote from the recently released WHO World Health Report (World Health Organization, 2004) since it clearly states the promise and the challenges ahead:

> Extending treatment opportunities needs a faster research process than is available through traditional notions of research. The nature of the HIV/AIDS epidemic is changing quickly in many countries—too quickly to be effectively countered through standard research processes, whose timeline is typically measured in years. In addition, many of the decisions on which research projects are to be funded and pursued are made by policy-makers at some distance from the problem. As a result, resources and efforts are invested in work that may have little or no relevance to actual implementation in the field. The public health community must rethink its definition of knowledge and the structure by which it is generated, shared and applied. The aims of knowledge management are to collect all

relevant information and intellectual capital into a common system, and provide equal access to that information, ensuring that it can be synthesized with local needs. Such a system enables members of the public health community to communicate directly with their peers on matters of mutual interest, such as effective practice in their own localities. The 3 by 5 goal prompts public health practitioners to share and exploit experiential knowledge in a much more direct way, for example through "communities of practice" - informal networks linking individuals and groups who share common professional interests and who benefit from frequent exchanges of knowledge through the Internet or other telecommunication methods. Progress in information and communication technologies and other learning systems such as communities of practice gives cause for optimism. Improved communication can spur a knowledge revolution that will particularly benefit poor countries and communities, through greater use of the Internet, e-mail and telephone, and better satellite and wireless technology. By whatever means, the promotion and improvement of learning systems at all levels should greatly assist the achievement of public health goals as well as helping to strengthen health systems in general. (p. 87)

REFERENCES

Britton, B. J., Evans, J. G., & Potter, J. M. (1998). Does the fly matter? The CRACKPOT study in evidence based trout fishing. *British Medical Journal, 317*, 1678–1680.

Clinicians for the Restoration of Autonomous Practice (CRAP) Writing Group (2002). EBM: Unmasking the ugly truth. *British Medical Journal, 325*, 1496–1498.

Davies, H. T. O., Nutley, S. M., & Smith, P. C. (2000). What works?: Evidence-based policy and practice in public services. Bristol: The Policy Press.

Davies, P. (2004). Is evidence-based government possible? Unpublished manuscript, London, England.

Gambrill, E. (1999). Evidence-based practice: An alternative to authority-based practice. *Families in Society: The Journal of Contemporary Human Services, 80*(4), 341.

Gibbs, L. E. (2003). Evidence-based practice for the helping professions: A practical guide with integrated multimedia. Pacific Grove, CA: Brooks/Cole-Thompson Learning.

Gibbs, L., & Gambrill, E. (2002). Evidence-based practice: Counterarguments to objections. *Research on Social Work Practice, 12*(3), 452–476.

Grahame-Smith, D. (1995). Evidence based medicine: Socratic dissent. *BMJ, 310*, 1126–1127.

Gray, J. A. M. (2001). Evidence-based healthcare (2nd ed.). New York: Churchill Livingstone.

Grayson, L., & Gomersall, A. (2003). A difficult business: finding the evidence for social science reviews. Unpublished manuscript, ESRC UK Centre for Evidence Based Policy and Practice, London, England, UK.

Macdonald, G. (1999). Evidence-based social care: Wheels off the runway? *Public Money & Management, 19*(1), 25–32.

Marshall, T. (1995). Letter to the editor. *The Lancet, 346,* 1171–1172.

Morgan, W. K. C. (1995). Letter to the editor. *The Lancet, 346,* 1172.

Moynihan, D.P. (1995. Rearranging flowers on the coffin [Congressional Record: December 12, 1995 (Senate)][Pages S18433–S18437] From the Congressional Record Online via GPO Access [wais.access.gpo.gov] [DOCID:cr12de95–110] retrieved April 23, 2004 from http://frwebgate3.access.gpo.gov/cgi-bin/waisgate.cgi?WAISdocID = 90341318293 + 0 + 0 + 0&WAISaction = retrieve

Mullen, E. (2004a). Evidence-based policy and practice: Implications for social work as a profession. *Sociale Interventie, 13*(4).

Mullen, E. J. (2004b). Facilitating practitioner use of evidence-based practice. In A. R. Roberts & K. Yeager (Eds.), *Evidence-Based Practice Manual: Research and Outcome Measures in Health and Human Services.* New York, NY: Oxford University Press.

Mullen, E. J., Shlonsky, A., Bledsoe, S. E., & Bellamy, J. L. (2005). From Concept to Implementation: Challenges Facing Evidence-based Social Work. *Evidence and Policy: A Journal of Debate, Research, and Practice, 1*(1).

Mullen, E. J., & Streiner, D. L. (2004). The evidence for and against evidence based practice. *Brief Treatment and Crisis Intervention, 4*(2).

Nutley, S. (2003). Bridging the policy/ research divide: Reflections and lessons from the UK. Unpublished manuscript. St. Andrews, KY.

Nutley, S., Walter, I., & Davies, H. (2002). From knowing to doing: A framework for understanding the evidence-to-practice agenda. Unpublished manuscript, St. Andrews, KY.

Roberts, A. R., & Yeager, K. R. (Eds.). (2004). *Evidence-Based Practice Manual: Research and Outcome Measures in Health and Human Services.* New York: Oxford University Press.

Sackett, D. L., Rosenberg, W. M. C., Gray, J. A. M., & et al. (1996). Evidence based medicine: What it is and what it isn't - It's about integrating individual clinical expertise and the best external evidence. *British Medical Journal, 312*(7023), 71–72.

Sackett, D. L., Straus, S. E., Richardson, W. S., Rosenberg, W., & Haynes, R. B. (2000). *Evidence-based medicine: How to practice and teach EBM* (2 ed.). New York: Churchill Livingstone.

Walker, R. (2001). Great expectations: Can social science evaluate New Labour's policies? *Evaluation, 7*(3), 305–330.

Webb, S. A. (2001). Some considerations on the validity of evidence-based practice in social work. *British Journal of Social Work, 31,* 57–79.

World Bank. (1999). World development report: Knowledge for development. Oxford: Oxford University Press.

World Health Organization (2001). The world health report 2001: Mental health new understandings, new hope. Geneva, Switzerland: World Health Organization.

World Health Organization (2004). The World Health Report 2000: Changing History. Geneva, Switzerland: World Health Organization.

Policy Barriers to the Employment of People Experiencing Psychiatric Disabilities

Janki Shankar, PhD

INTRODUCTION

Successive Australian governments since the late eighties have increasingly pursued policies aimed at stemming the growing numbers of citizens who are claiming the Disability Support Pension. The previous Labor government in 1990–91, introduced the Disability Reform Program (DRP) to improve the participation of individuals with disabilities in employment, particularly those with significant disabilities (Baume and

Kay, 1995). The DRP had special provisions for people with psychiatric disabilities. Before its introduction individuals with psychiatric disabilities were seen as the responsibility of state governments, not the Commonwealth, and were not eligible for Commonwealth funded employment and training services available to individuals with other disabilities (Whitford et al., 1993). The DRP granted this group access to mainstream training, rehabilitation, and other disability employment support services. However, access to programs cannot result in successful employment outcomes unless the programs meet the specific needs of the individuals. Evaluation of the DRP indicated that it had failed to meet the employment needs of those with severe disabilities, and this included psychiatric disabilities (Baume and Kay, 1995).

The Liberal Coalition Government, which was elected to office in 1996, has initiated a series of welfare reforms to move those with disabilities into employment. This article argues that although work is of benefit for many individuals with psychiatric disability, the current policy changes are unlikely to improve their employment outcomes. Current policies will not only diminish their chances for employment, but will also reduce their chances of recovery.

I first present an overview of three policy changes (since the takeover by the Liberal Government in 1996) that have impacted on the employment outcomes of this group. These are: (1) competitive tendering of employment services; (2) policy of mutual obligation; and (3) outcome-driven-assessment–focused funding policies. Second, I present a discussion of the role of current policies in shaping employment outcomes and recovery.

RECENT WELFARE REFORM POLICIES FOR PEOPLE WITH DISABILITIES

Competitive Tendering of Employment Services

One of the first major reforms undertaken by the Liberal Government was to restructure employment services along market lines. It sought to achieve this by establishing a separation between the policy and service delivery units of two major departments that had the joint responsibility of providing employment and income support services. These two departments were the Department of Education, Employment, Training and Youth Affairs (DEETYA) and the Department of Social Security (DSS). The government dismantled the service delivery arm of DEETYA, namely, the Commonwealth Employment Service (CES), an entity which provided employment services such as job training, job matching and limited case-management services to all job seekers.

In 1999 the CES was replaced with Job Network: a national network of private and nongovernment agencies which now compete in a quasi-marketplace for contracts to deliver services to the unemployed. Corporations and nonprofit community and religious organizations within the Job Network receive funding for the provision of various levels of support for job seekers, including Job matching, Job Search Training and Intensive Assistance (Department of Employment, Workplace Relations and Small Business, 2000).

The Job Network was combined with a new agency, Centrelink, and together they have responsibility for employment services, social security payments, and a few other Commonwealth payments. The former Department of Social Security (DSS) was reduced to a policy unit, the Department of Family and Community services (DFaCs), which functions as a purchaser of services from Centrelink. With the establishment of Job Network and Centrelink, the Government made a major shift from its role of provider of services to purchaser and contractor. However, the Government maintains control through its monopoly position as a dispenser of contracts and supplier of clients. With employment services now contracted out through a competitive tendering process, it was expected that costs would be significantly reduced.

The Government maintains that competition among employment service providers (including disability employment providers) will provide "choice" to consumers, encourage innovation in service delivery, and improve outcomes. Although the government has widely heralded the "success" of its competition-based employment service delivery system, there is already evidence that the Job Network has not been particularly successful in placing disadvantaged jobseekers in employment (Eardley Abello, & Macdonald, 2001). Nevertheless, with the Job Network firmly in place the government over a period of 4 years from 1996 had cut its expenditure on labor market programs and case-management services by $AUS1.8 billion (Ranald, 2002).

The Policy of Mutual Obligation

The most recent ideological shift of the current Government towards recipients of the Disability Support Pension is expressed through the policy of "mutual obligation." Till recently people with disabilities were not required to undertake activities such as rehabilitation, training, and job search as a condition of disability support payments. The government claimed that this was an "unintended incentive" that was built into the DSP and because of which welfare dependency among the disabled had increased significantly. Changes outlined in the 2002–2003 Common-wealth budget are designed to ensure that continued eligibility to income support for all recipients, whether with a disability or not, would be based on their undertaking activities such as rehabilitation, training and job search, or work-for-the-dole scheme. Individuals on income support payments who do not cooperate with this policy are at risk of having their payments suspended.

In adopting this policy, the Government can be seen to have taken a paternalistic approach to individuals with a disability, implying that they are dependent, and lacking in competence, initiative, and motivation. The role of the state, then, has been to assume the position of a "wise and firm father figure" who knows what is in the best interests of his citizens, how they should achieve their aims, and what pressures should be applied to ensure they conform (Mead, 1997). Though the government claims that employment outcomes of individuals with disabilities will be improved through the enforcement of this policy, recent research already shows that it is failing to meet the needs of those with the greatest barriers to employment (Ziguras et al, 2003).

Outcome-Driven-Assessment–Focused Funding Policies

In the current system all jobseekers can access the Job Network. However, those who identify as having disabilities have to undergo assessments of their work capacity and employment assistance needs. Two measures are currently used to assess these, namely, the Work Ability Tables (WATs) and the Job Support Classification Index (JSCI). The purpose of these assessments is to stream people into appropriate services and allocate case based funding.

The WATs is based on the assumption that a small number of 'core work abilities' are fundamental for successful participation in the workforce. A cut-off score is used to stream individuals into services. Those scoring less than the cut-off are directed to the Job Network system which provides three levels of support: Job Matching (Flex1), Job Search Training (Flex 2), and Intensive Assistance (Flex 3). Those scoring above the cut-off on the WATs are considered to have significant disability-related barriers to employment. These are streamed into the DFaCS which receives case based funding for providing supported and open employment services (Disability Industry Reference Group, 1999). The JSCI scores are used to determine the level of employment assistance required by the individual and to allocate case based funding. This system, in principle, allows those assessed as having greater needs to be allocated more resources. In practice, this means the service provider receives funding at a higher level for these individuals, even though the number and type of services offered to the "client" is not legislated for, but decided upon by the provider. The Government claims that the policy of assessing needs and allocating funds achieves better outcomes for job seekers with disabilities, as it is a system based on the principles of enhanced access and choice, an equitable funding model, and a more flexible and innovative service delivery system (Disability Employment Services, 1997). However, a preliminary evaluation of this funding model for individuals with psychiatric disabilities has indicated that though their participation rate in employment programs has increased, it has not been accompanied by a commensurate improvement in employment outcomes (Department of Family and Community Services, Casebased funding Trial Phase 1 Statistical update March 2001). The Government plans to improve outcomes by further "refining the assessment tools."

The above discussion has provided an overview of three recent policies that aim to improve the employment prospects of individuals with disabilities. Next, I discuss the role of these policies in shaping employment outcomes and recovery for people with psychiatric disabilities.

Role of Current Policies in Shaping Employment Outcomes and Recovery

Several studies have shown that individuals with psychiatric disabilities can be successful in employment if they have appropriate support and that employment can improve their quality of life (Drake et al., 1999; Meuser 1997; Van Dongen, 1996). It is also known that people with psychiatric disabilities are a heterogeneous group at various stages of recovery from the illness and that not all will be ready or suited for open employment. Therefore, a variety of work options (such as transitional employment or group business enterprises), must be available to sustain their hope, motivation and capacity for work Bachrach (1992). Studies on rehabilitation and recovery from mental illness demonstrate that individuals with psychiatric disabilities, who are recovering need to experience a sense of control over their situation and the rehabilitation process. Control over one's own rehabilitation process increases commitment, involvement, and motivation to achieve goals, all of which are important for recovery (Deegan, 1988, 1996). Factors that can sustain people's motivation to persist with vocational rehabilitation are a genuine interest in gaining employment, the choice that the program offers to try out their capacity for work, active involvement in the process of setting work goals and activities, and the awareness that they can withdraw from the program at any time without penalty or loss of entitlement to the pension.

Though the concept of "recovery" from mental illness has been variously defined, recovery is oriented towards regaining one's self esteem, being able to make choices, establishing meaningful relationships with others, and performing social roles (Deegan, 1996; Townsend & Glasser, 2003). Recovery from mental illness, however, is not a linear process and individuals may move back and forth in their attempts to recover.

Employment is an important factor that can be linked to recovery. Research shows that employment can provide meaning and purpose to one's life, increase personal empowerment, and help individuals recover their self esteem and confidence (Young & Ensing, 1999; Torrey & Wyzik, 2000; Provencher, Gregg, Mearl, & Mueser, 2002). A factor that is crucial for recovery is the relationship between the professional helper and the individual who is recovering. Professionals in rehabilitation need to convey a sense of hope, be nonjudgemental in their approach, and not make individuals feel they are lazy, lacking in motivation, or "low functioning" (Deegan, 1988).

The policy of mutual obligation requires individuals with psychiatric disabilities to undertake various activities in return for the pension. This neither increases employment outcomes nor enhances prospects of recovery for a number of reasons. First of all there is an assumption that these individuals must be compelled towards work because they are, by nature, lacking in the initiative and motivation and prefer to be dependent on public income support. Research evidence challenges this view however, as it shows that individuals with psychiatric disabilities have often made several attempts to gain employment but have been thwarted by their illness and barriers in the social environment (e.g., Shankar & Collyer, 2003).

Second, the policy of mutual obligation infringes on the rights of those with psychiatric disabilities to maintain control over their recovery process, and to exercise "choice" about whether or not to participate in rehabilitation. Participation in rehabilitation must be based on a genuine interest to gain employment. Participation that is driven by fear, such as the loss of the pension or by the lack of appropriate support for the family or the community, is not likely to result in a successful outcome.

Third the policy of mutual obligation is at risk of jeopardizing the relationship between the professional helper and the individual with disabilities, because it enforces a system where professionals control the rehabilitation process. Rather than working in partnership, professionals within this policy context, can become "policing" agents, with rights to use punitive measures (such as imposing penalties on those who breach contracts), to control resources, and pursue narrowly defined outcomes in a market driven system. Consequently, those with psychiatric disabilities, who are already one of the most powerless groups in society, are further disempowered and will be offered little hope of recovery.

With respect to the assessment of work capacity, studies have shown that situational assessments may be the best means currently available for assessing the work abilities of individuals with psychiatric disabilities (Rehabilitation Services Administration, Office of Special Education, US Department of Education, 1995; Anthony and Jansen, 1984; Tashjian, Hayward, Stoddard, & Kraus, 1989). Situational assessments are skill-focused, rather than impairment-focused, and can be completed by the assessor (rehabilitation professional and the workplace supervisor) based on their direct observation of performance in the actual work setting over a period of time. They can identify specific areas of strength and difficulty early in the course of the program, thus providing the opportunity for improvement. However situational assessments are often time and labor intensive and need vocationally trained staff and work settings (MacDonald, Rogers, & Anthony, 2001).

Although situational assessments hold greater promise than other forms of assessment, even these may be unable to address the day to day fluctuations in functioning, or the hidden heterogeneity, each of which are characteristic of psychiatric disability. This calls into question the predictive validity of the quick, cross sectional assessments of work ability and employment assistance (WATs and JSCI) that are currently used for the purposes of streaming individuals into services and allocating case based funding. The use of these assessments for individuals with psychiatric disability is associated with several risks.

First, both these measures (WATs and JSCI), are largely based on the self-reports of individuals. Many individuals may not be aware of their work related difficulties or may not want to disclose their difficulties because of the fear of discrimination. Others may not be fully aware of the association between the illness and the problems they face. (which is not surprising, given the fundamental indeterminacy of psychiatric diagnosis: see for example, Fox 2000). These factors can lead to the under reporting of disabilities and to referrals to services which cannot provide the appropriate form and level of support. This not only will result in poor employment outcomes, but can lead to individuals leaving programs before completion, suspension of their benefits, and the associated risks of greater dependence on family or homelessness.

Second, the high drop-out rates from employment programs and the low employment outcomes of those with psychiatric disabilities may reinforce public perceptions that they are poor candidates for employment. Furthermore, although benefit recipients are expected to submit to assessments of their work ability, and participate in rehabilitation, job training or other work related activities, there is no guarantee they will be placed into jobs nor receive appropriate training. Thus the current system not only sets up individuals for failure, but may add to poor community attitudes and self stigmatization (Petersen et al., 2002). In the current outcome-driven employment services market, such stereotyping can further jeopardize an individual's chances of gaining employment. For individuals with psychiatric disabilities, this system can intensify feelings of hopelessness, a condition that is not conducive to recovery.

Third the policy's focus on the assessment of impairments and disabilities reflects an uncritical acceptance of the medical model of disability. This places emphasis on the individual's capacity for skill building and performance and obscures the extent to which the social environment provides a range of obstacles. An adherence to the medical model ensures that resources are directed towards refining assessment tools and measures rather than addressing the social factors that shape employment outcomes.

Social Factors That Shape Employment Outcomes

The social barriers to employment are posed by employers, family networks, and treatment providers. Our experience suggests that although employers may accept people with psychiatric disabilities for placement in their organizations, they may still not offer them employment for several reasons (Shankar & Collyer, 2003). These include lack of confidence about giving negative feedback in case they "upset" the individual and apprehensions about their own ability to handle future, possible crisis situations or respond appropriately when changes have been noted in the employee's behavior. Such concerns highlight the stigma associated with mental illness and the lack of information among employers about the nature of psychiatric disability. If employers are to offer employment and be supportive resources must be directed towards their education and training, and they need to be provided with ongoing professional support. Studies show that the more aware and knowledgeable employers are about mental illness and psychiatric disability, the more likely it is that they will hire these individuals (Akabas, 1994).

Family networks and treatment professionals also need education and support. Family members comprise the largest component of the networks of those with psychiatric disabilities, and play a significant role in their lives. However, families may, understandably, fail to be committed to their relative's employment goals when their own needs for professional support, respite, information and involvement are not met. Treatment providers can also play a role in shaping employment outcomes. Research indicates that many tend to be overprotective, paternalistic and hold conservative views about their client's capacity for employment (Nicholson, 1994; Graffam and Nacarella, 1994). Thus some of the significant social barriers to employment may come from within the mental health system itself.

IMPLICATIONS AND CONCLUSION

This report shows that successful employment outcomes for people with disabilities depend not on the individual alone, but on the cooperative efforts of many differently placed individuals and organizations. In turn, these actors function to provide support within a broad array of government policies which shape and steer programs and services. The current policy context however, is based on market principles with its goals of competition, cost efficiency, and financial incentives. Here the individual is treated as a market consumer rather than a citizen, and the medical model is adopted as the means to provide services (Sherry, 2002). Although the Government claims that competition and outcome-based funding will enhance "choice," improve the quality of services, encourage innovativeness and equity, in practice this system may force employment service agencies to compete rather than cooperate with one another for the "best clients," that is, for those who are less disabled, whose disabilities are predictable, who need minimum employment support, and who tend to achieve "quick outcomes." There is little room in this system for those with severe psychiatric disabilities who may be successful at work but need innovative and challenging approaches to employment support.

If Government is really committed to improving employment outcomes for individuals with psychiatric disabilities, it must consider funding for rehabilitation and employment programs from an investment, rather than short-term, outcome perspective. Such a perspective will encourage the development of innovative approaches to providing employment support, the setting-up of a range of vocational options for individuals at various stages of recovery, and the involvement of all members of the network in these initiatives. It would also review the competitive market approach to the employment services sector and establish cooperative initiatives between employment services for sharing specialized knowledge and skills in the area of vocational rehabilitation. Finally, it would have to examine the medical model of disability and the way this has hampered efforts at establishing constructive working partnerships between individuals with a disability and their treatment professionals, and between the employment services and the treatment system.

REFERENCES

Akabas, S. H. (1994). Workplace responsiveness: Key employer characteristics in support of job maintenance for people with mental illness. *Psychosocial Rehabilitation Journal, 17*(3), 91–101.

Anthony, W. A., & Jansen, M. (1984). Predicting the vocational capacity of the chronically mentally ill: Research and policy implications. *American Psychologist, 39*, 537–544

Bachrach, L. L. (1992). Psychosocial rehabilitation and psychiatry in the care of long-term patients. *The American Journal of Psychiatry, 149*, 11.

Baume, P., & Kay, K. (1995). *Working solution.* Report of the strategic review of the commonwealth disability services program. Canberra: Commonwealth of Australia.

Department of Family and Community Services Report (2001). *Casebased Funding Trial-Phase One Statistical Update.* www.facs.gov.au

Deegan, P. E. (1988). Recovery: The lived experience of rehabilitation. *Psychosocial Rehabilitation Journal, 11*(4), 11–19.

Deegan, P. E. (1996). Recovery as a journey of the heart. *Psychiatric Rehabilitation Journal, 19*(3), 91–97.

Department of Employment, Workplace Relations and Small Business (2000). *Job network evaluation, stage one: implementation and market development.* EPPB Report (1/2000), Canberra: Evaluation and Program Performance Branch, DEWRSB.

Department of Family and Community Services, Case based Funding Trial 1 statistical Update at March 2001. www.facs.gov.au

Disability Industry Reference Group (1999). *The effectiveness of the new employment assessment and streaming arrangements for job seekers with disabilities.* www.facs.gov.au.

Drake, R. E., McHugo, G. J., Bebout, R. R., Becker, D. R., Harris, M., Bond, G. R., & Quimby, E. (1999). A randomized clinical trial of supported employment for inner-city patients with severe mental disorders. *Archives of General Psychiatry, 56,* 627–633.

Eardley, T., Abello, D., & Macdonald, H. (2001). *Is the job network benefiting the disadvantaged job seekers? Preliminary evidence from a study of non-profit employment services.* Discussion Paper No 111. Sydney: Social Policy Research Centre, University of New South Wales.

Fox, R. (2000). Medical uncertainty revisited. In G. Albrecht, R. Fitzpatrick, & S. Scrimshaw (Eds.). *The Handbook of Social Studies in Health and Medicine*, pp. 409–425. London: Sage.

Graffam, J., & Nacarella, L. (1994). *National Evaluation Project.* Canberra: Commonwealth Department of Human Services and Health, Disability Services Program.

MacDonald-Wilson, K., Rogers, E. S., & Anthony, W. A. (2001). Unique issues in assessing work function among individuals with psychiatric disabilities. *Journal of Occupational Rehabilitation, 11*(3), 217–231.

Mead, L. M. (1997). The rise of paternalism. In L. M. Mead (Ed.), *The new paternalism: supervisory approaches to poverty.* Washington DC: Brookings Institution.

Meuser, K. T., Becker, D. R., & Torrey, W. C. (1997). Recent advances in psychiatric rehabilitation for patients with severe mental illness. *Harvard Review of Psychiatry, 5,* 123–137.

Nicholson, P. (1994). *Building bridges to work – that work.* Mental Health Services Conference, September.

Petersen, A., Kokanovic, R., & Hansen, S. (2002). Consumerism and mental health care in a culturally diverse society. In S. Henderson & A. Petersen (Eds.), *Consuming Health: The Commodification of Health Care*, pp. 121–139. London: Routledge.

Provencher, H. L., Gregg, R., Mead, S., & Mueser, T. M. (2002). The role of work in the recovery of persons with psychiatric disabilities. *Psychiatric Rehabilitation Journal, 26*(2), 132–144.

Ranald, P. (2002) Where are the jobs in the Job Network? Competitive Tendering of Employment Services, In P. Fairbrother, M. Paddon, & J. Teicher (Eds.), *Privatization, Globalization and Labor, Studies from Australia*, pp. 158–160. Annandale, NSW: Federation Press.

Rehabilitation Services Administration (1995). *The provision of vocational rehabilitation services to individuals who have severe mental illness: Program administration review.* (Final Report). Washington DC: Office of Special Education and Rehabilitation Services, U.S. Department of Education.

Shankar, J., & Collyer, F. M. (2003). Vocational rehabilitation of people with mental illness: The need for a broader approach. *Australian e-Journal of Mental Health (AeJAMH), 2,* Issue 2, 1–13.

Sherry, M. (2002). Welfare reform and disability policy in Australia. *Just Policy, 28,* 3–11.

Tashjian, M. D., Hayward, B. J., Stoddard, S., Kraus, L. (1989). *Best practice study of vocational rehabilitation services to severely mentally ill persons. Volume 1, Study findings.* Washington DC: Policy Study Associates.

Torrey, W. C., & Wyzik, P. (2000). The Recovery vision as a service improvement guide for community mental health centre providers. *Community Mental Health Journal, 36*(2), 209–216.

Townsend, W., & Glasser, N. (2003). Recovery: the heart and soul of treatment. *Psychosocial Rehabilitation Journal, 27* (1), 83–86.

Van Dongen, C. J. (1996). Quality of life and self esteem in working and non working persons with mental illness. *Community Mental Health Journal, 32*(6), 535–547.

Whitford, H. A., Behan, S., Leitch, E., McGowan, T., Macloed, B., Spencer, D., Fleming, T., & Solomon, S. (1993). *Help where help is needed: continuity of care for people with chronic mental illness*. Issues Paper No. 5. Canberra: National Health Strategy.

Young, S. L., & Ensing, D. S. (1999). Exploring recovery from the perspective of people with psychiatric disabilities. *Psychiatric Rehabilitation Journal, 22*, 219–231.

Ziguras, S., Dufty, G. & Considine, M. (2003). *Much obliged: Disadvantaged job seekers' experiences of the mutual obligation regime*. Fitzroy, Victoria: Brotherhood of St. Laurence.

Index

Printed and bound by CPI Group (UK) Ltd, Croydon, CR0 4YY

17/10/2024

01775695-0001